THE KAMASUTRA EXPERIENCE

WITH ALL THE BEST SEX POSITIONS

Lawrence Iulius

Contents

Chapter One

INTRODUCTION

This is A final decision, but it creates a lot of possibilities to get the best difference. He believes that woman does not mean love with will. This is part of our story with Cubic Nephrosis and Grass ESC. Have you ever driven someone? Otherwise, it is unacceptable.These fears are perhaps positive motivations because all concentrations with results occur between times. However, it's different every time, you can try different options, but people are looking! They are the best of all! For most men, length is an important issue at some point. Now he knows best. Most men are considered. In many cases, young people refer to the next sixth meeting.So, they extend it as long as possible. It usually takes 10-10 minutes to resolve the climax, which for some reason is not necessarily a source of love. So, in this case, we offer some very important alternatives for you to choose the time and moment. At the end of this study, more than 70 people are playing to improve their safety. It contains conditions to ensure full participation. It's a nearby commercial hotel - the hotel has amenities unlike other methods you can lay out at special rates. There is only one chance to suspend because there is a gap. You can also discuss things without scheduling a meeting.It is better to have a free and quiet place. In this sense, we offer the best with the best opportunities to spend free time during sex.I think if you have a Romanian they know exactly when you have sex and not intimacy. ▨▨▨▨▨▨

▨▨▨▨▨. That why is because of respect, many will you do sexual positions enjoy but prevent of the the springs mattress squeak, bars of the the bed sound, or even, sometimes, someone between you and the language catch act. Ask, this product may be available - you can avoid tax problems and different items you need. We know we love it, so thank you, it's great, but it's great, but it's hard. Some of the broader possibilities of expression suggest that perhaps it is not a decision, but rather a separate decision. It is better to make sure that they end at the same time and at different times. The Kafir was very different even in his love. You can see many of them, love them and the unexplored sixth world. They try to link their great pleasure with love, which is why they have entered the list of new projects .Every time from the most difficult place to the most popular. But the truth is that no mantra can ever evoke situations, confuse the mind and find something new. In this case, you can learn more about what you want. This new feature is based on new parameters. So, there are many things to consider, but there are some important aspects that we rarely know about. Our choices are short because the pros and cons of these choices are some of the things you need to consider. Se vi always devas eviti krei kaj provi new things, profitu či tion. Even, ▢▢▢▢▢▢▢ ▢▢▢▢▢, comfort zone, a wor wout with wor gourestrustrustrut worexual sexual e t worexual e t worexual e rexual thexual thexual thexual thexual thexual thexual thexual thexual thexual thexual thexual thexual thexual e t worexual thexual sexual sexual sexual sexut worexut e e t e balance partner.

Chapter Two

Various proven sex positions

Different types Sexual posesInitially, you need to know that the classification of sexual situations depends on the following patterns.Man-to-face man: This mode is common between couples and is characterized by face-to-face communication. A standard aspect of this type is an advertising pose in which a woman is presented with her legs open. A man is lying on the ground and can use this position for anal or vaginal intercourse. At one stage, a woman can hang her leg over the edge of the stage or lift it from the ceiling in a pose often known as the butterfly pose. You can do the same while kneeling. In another version, the woman can place her legs on the man's shoulders. Straightening, the penis moves down to rub the vagina with an upward movement of the penis. In addition, the woman lies with her legs raised to her head or close to her ears. Then the male grabs the ankles or lifts the pair and lies on the female for a long time. Most partners prefer this style because it is emotionally and physically nutritious.Eye Contact: In this mode, screens can read facial expressions and keep eye contact for maximum enjoyment. Masala: In this mode, husband and wife keep their hands free and can kiss, kiss and stimulate the clitoris.Dominant man: space creates concentration, man dominates the soul and rhythm, speed and level of penetration. Relaxation: Women prefer this position while lying on the bed.Dilation: Varieties in this position are best for dilation because they make a deep penetration that ejaculates close to the cervix. Communication: When a couple tries on new clothes, body language and direct comments increase.Next: Even after sex, the man hugs, hugs and kisses her easily. Uncontrollable Ejaculation: Men with this condition cannot control their bodies because they are busy and constantly moving forward. That's why they can't stop ejaculating. Incomplete penetration: This is common, especially if the woman has a wide waist. Thighs can prevent deep penetration. Less stimulus: Most variations of this pose require the woman to place her legs higher than the man's arms or chest. This condition causes the penis to go down and up through the clitoris, causing little or no stimulation. Reverse Penetration: Most of these styles are suitable for both anal and vaginal sex. This pattern is sometimes described as a dog style, although there are many variations. In this style, the woman lies down and holds her upper body horizontally to penetrate from behind. Similarly, a man can bend his body while lifting his hips to achieve full penetration. By bending the knees, the penetrating partner can place his feet in addition to the partner and rise as high as possible to maintain penetration. A husband can put his hands on his wife's back so that she doesn't fall forward. When a man extends his hands, a woman can also kneel. Another variation of this style is the spoon, where the pair is positioned in the same direction, kneeling, standing or lying on the bed. For maximum stimulation and penetration, it is recommended to place a pillow under the woman's pelvis. Men find this style satisfying and pleasurable because it gives a piercing look when their partner rises and falls. This technique allows them to print in care and we know the service that shows the channel.ben efitsHands Free: This position allows both parties to use their hands to further stimulate each other. Full sense: for men who rejoice in the gentleness of the donkey. It creates a pleasant atmosphere that captivates the couple. Fertility: The deep penetration associated with this condition makes it easier for a woman to get pregnant because it traps sperm near the cervix. Sound effects: The soft body around the woman's hips makes a rhythmic sound in response to your pushes. evil-Eye Contact: Penetration begins from behind, which means no eye contact unless the woman withdraws. This makes it difficult to understand your partner's feelings. Possible injury: If people try to hit hard and miss with the vagina, they can damage the penis - this position also nar-rows the vagina and allows the man to acciden-tally hit it.Women's Top: This style is designed to penetrate the anus and vagina. Other names: shepherdess, shepherdess or woman from above. The most characteristic feature of this style is that the man lies on his back and the listeners sit or lie on them. This technique gives the woman the opportunity to look in the opposite direction, colloquially called inversion. They can bend in front of a man and touch only the genitals. In the lateral coitus position, the man lies on his back, the recipient turns slightly, legs apart. This style has mission-like features, in which case the woman is responsible. Above, the woman is not as unchained as she is penetrated. A cow culminates faster than a guy without effort. As a couple, they can change roles, get intimate, and share what works best for you. Fit is a general indicator of how well the style suits you.benefits·

Eye Contact: Like the man above, partners can make direct eye contact and read facial expressions. · Training partners can use their hands to caress and stimulate each other's genitals.· Access to the clitoris: This position allows the man to reach the clitoris and rub it. · Visual stimulation: Men with this disease can see a reality that stimulates their sexual feelings.· Controlled Ejaculation: This is the best article for men who want to control their ejaculation. Due to the lack of pressure and effort, a man can sometimes control his passion.· Adjustable rhythm: women from above control the rhythm, speed and depth of penetration. Pregnancy: Women like this pose during pregnancy because it reduces pressure on the abdomen. Similarly, nursing mothers can use it to control all aspects of sex. · Relaxation for men: as the woman gets up, the man under her relaxes, and the penis remains strongly vertical. This is an ideal position for men recovering from illness. evilFatigue. For women, this situation is exhausting because she is not doing all the work necessary.· Withdrawal: Men complain that the penis needs to move, especially if the penis is short. Likewise, men with erectile dysfunction will find this place less desirable. To improve this condition, you need to have and maintain a strong erection. · Passive people: For people who think they are in control, this position violates control. He lets them watch as the girl resumes the session. However, they may try to raise their hips to participate.Sit and Kneel: Showdown is the most common style of this genre and there are no words to describe it. This technique usu-ally consists of the woman sitting on the man and gently grasping his erogenous zones. Alternative-ly, the man may sit on a chair while the receiver performs the lap dance. When a man looks at a woman's back, it can be done in the opposite position. Partners can even sit on the sofa bed.

The female sits upright on the mating towers. For short places, the man can kneel and the woman lies on her back with the ankles on her shoulders. Walking works best when you don't have enough room to move or stretch. For example, you can transport and your caravan does not have a bathroom, so it uses the space provided on the seats. This is a relaxed style because both partners are compatible. He makes it work with you and moves only the important part for good sex. benefits·· Less noise: due to the proximity of the genitals, the position requires less pressure, so relative silence.Location This approach ensures that the penis is in the correct L position in this position, as is the sheath.· Touch: When couples sit or kneel against each other, they increase visual stimulation and prolong kissing and tenderness. evil· Fitness required: Long knees can be problematic for some couples and make it difficult to hold the pose.Standing: If you want to have sex while standing, you can add different types. You can have face-to-face vaginal sex. A woman can allow penetration by slightly opening her hips. If one of the pair is low, he may wear high heels or stand on a ladder. Abundance is more reliable, especially if a woman leans against the wall. This rack supports both sides and is best used in vertical spaces such as bathrooms or bedrooms. A woman can stand with her arms around a man's neck and legs. This style exposes the vagina and anus to a vertical penis. Initially, this can be done by lying on the bed and allowing the man to place his elbows below his knees. He decides to get in, get up and take her. During anal action, a woman can look at a man and take different standing and half-standing positions. For example, they can slide their hips and place their hands on the platform.

Advantages

· Fast: This is the best mode if you want to do it fast or don't have time to go to the camera .Role Play: This part allows the man to change roles because both are in the same position. Body Connection: The standing position improves the relationship with the whole body, especially if couples are completely naked.· Leaning: When a woman leans against a wall, she leans on both sides. In this way, a person can find an opportunity for deeper penetration.· Warning: In this mode, both parties can kiss and be kissed, especially if they face each other. evil· Shorter partners: Chairs can be uncomfortable for members of different sizes. The genitals may not line up, which requires a change in the couple's position. · Planning Required: While practicing this position, partners should plan ahead. It helps a person not to fall when he uses his passion, energy and aggression. · Physical condition: When one partner needs support, the other must be prepared for the heavy responsibility of maintaining his weight. A woman must bear the weight of a man and be able to balance at the waist. Balance is important in this situation.15 best sex positions and how to do themMissionary 180: This position reverses the traditional missionary but requires human flexibility! A woman should lie on her back and spread her legs. Then the man should be in the upper part, but the head should be directed towards the feet and the feet should be on both sides of his body. When taking the position, the man must carefully push the penis down and penetrate the sexual partner. Sit comfortably and press up and down.Security CouncilThis pose requires a very flexible male penis. Before joining, make sure you are comfortable! There is a risk that he will hang his limb and pull the ligaments. If you feel severe pain, leave the position and find something more comfortable. When starting work, a woman should be careful not to squeeze the penis. Self-Bumper This is an intense sexual position that allows for deep penetration. Great if you need a G-spot timer to culminate. Again, this position requires penile flexibility, so make sure the man is comfortable in this position. Start with the woman lying on her stomach with her legs apart and her legs straight. A man should lie on his stomach, open his legs and stretch them. You have to look in the opposite direction. Then the man turns to his partner so that his hips are on her hips. Do this until your penis enters your wife's vagina. Then slowly enter.safety tipsThis position requires the flexibility of the penis. If you want to know if the penis is flexible enough, press it.

Gradually pull out the penis. If the penis points directly into the ground without causing pain, it should be fine, but you should always be careful. A woman must be silent when a man enters. Wait until the woman finds the most comfortable position and angle to push without injuring herself.

Human These pitfalls are different advertising situations. Let the woman lie down on the bed, and let the man lie down on her. When he starts pushing, the woman can wrap her legs around him and control the speed and speed of intercourse. Great if you want pure sex. For the best stimulus, you can make small movements like flexible on your back. Surround the legs around the man moves it too fast!Security tipsThese conditions can cause a lot of stress at the bottom of a woman, so make sure he offers a pillow or wearer! Ask if your partner is always comfortable and painless if you have something to say, because you are ashamed, please!The comic contact with the closer and face face. One leg should stand on the bed and the other on the man's hand while the woman kisses his shoulder and back. Then you have to penetrate carefully. Once installed, a great image that looks amazing! However, this requires some resistance.safety tipsThis position requires the flexibility of the penis. Otherwise, there is a risk of tightening a person's suspension ligaments! If you want to know if the penis is flexible enough, press it. Gradually pull out the penis. If the penis points directly into the ground without causing pain, it should be fine, but you should always be careful. A woman must be calm when a man enters her for the first time and inserts his penis into her vagina. Wait until the woman finds the most comfortable position and angle to push without injuring herself.The floor chair requires the man to sit on the bed with his legs outstretched and his hands behind his head to support his weight. You should bend over and bend your elbows slightly. A woman must lie on a pillow in front of him and wrap her arms around his legs. Then you can shake your hips back and forth and start having sex. This is an incredible position for intense penetration to stimulate the G-spot. Security tip-sThese conditions can cause a lot of stress in the lower part of the woman, so be sure to make a pillow or pillow! Ask if your partner is always comfortable and painless if you have something to say, because you are ashamed, please!This is difficult because the corridor should be comfortable in a closed area. The man must lean on the wall and move to the ground to touch his feet on the wall. A woman has to stand up and carry her own weight. Your legs should hang and you can push. Perfect for adventure and exciting sex!safety tipsThe husband must make sure that he can support his wife's weight and not slip and fall completely on the floor. Similarly, a woman should carry her own weight as much as she can. The rotating support should start lying on your back with your legs apart. Ask your partner to stand on all fours between your legs. Then the woman would have to stand up and put her arms around her chest to support herself. Then you should slowly lift your legs so that your feet are on the floor. This is a great pose for deep penetration and G-spot stimulation!safety tipsThis position requires upper body strength. He needs to make sure he is firmly attached to his partner during the push.

SPIDER You should start looking at each other. The female should rise to the partner's knees and allow penetration. The legs should be bent from the sides, the man should do the same. First the female should lie down, then slowly the male, until both heads are on the bed. Now move slowly and quietly. This is a great choice for slow sex to increase arousal before climax, a great choice if you have a lot of time. safety tipsThis position requires the flexibility of the penis. Otherwise, there is a risk of tightening a person's suspension ligaments! If you want to know if the penis is flexible enough, press it. Gradually pull out the penis. If the penis goes straight to the floor without causing pain, it should be fine, but you should always be careful. A woman must be calm when a man enters her for the first time and inserts his penis into her vagina. Wait until the woman finds the most comfortable position and angle to push without injuring herself. The speed limiter should lie down and spread his legs. The male should enter from behind. The benefit of this situation is that everything can be warm and accelerated. If you have a little difficult or fast, it's the highest level!Security tipsThese conditions can cause a lot of stress in the lower part of the woman, so be sure to make a pillow or pillow! Ask if your partner is always comfortable and painless if you have something to say, because you are ashamed, please!A successful curve must sit on the area of the man's foot. A woman should sit with her legs spread on both sides and kneel on the penis. After penetration, you can lie down until you can stand. This position can give a woman a huge climax and a man can stimulate her breasts and nipples during intercourse.safety tipsThis position requires the flexibility of the penis. Otherwise, there is a risk of tightening a person's suspension ligaments! If you want to know if the penis is flexible enough against the wall. Gradually pull out the penis. If the penis goes straight to the floor without causing pain, it should be fine, but you should always be careful.A woman must be silent when a man enters her for the first time and inserts his penis into her vagina. Wait until the woman finds the most comfortable position and angle to push without injuring herself.The butterfly girl should lie on her back, legs apart, side by side. Man must be on the ground, but keep his feet. After penetration, the man should relax his hips, not push. This is a difficult position to master, practice is needed!safety tipsThis position requires the flexibility of the penis. Otherwise, there is a risk of tightening a person's suspension ligaments! If you want to know if the penis is flexible enough, press it. Gradually pull out the penis. If the penis goes straight to the floor without causing pain, it should be fine, but you should always be careful. A woman must be calm when a man enters her for the first time and inserts his penis into her vagina. Wait until the woman finds the most comfortable position and angle to push without injuring herself. In this wheelchair position, starting in a dog position, ask the woman to place her forearm on a pillow. His partner should bend his knees and kneel behind him to make sure. After entering, he must hold his legs, slowly lift them and stand up. This level is great if you try and laugh! Otherwise, it is too difficult and not worth trying. safety tipsDuring the push, the man should bend his knees slightly. If one of you feels uncomfortable in this situation, let the other know and try something else! This is not for you. Wise saddle. In this position, the male lies on his back, legs bent and separated, the immobile part while the male lies on the ground. A woman has to slide between her legs, almost straight to her body. To support yourself, place one hand on your chest and the other on your leg. This position depends on the woman swinging back and forth until she feels she has reached the G-spot. The best thing in this situation is that a woman has full control. So, if you have to reach the vagina, stimulating a G-spot-one of the best.Security tipsThese conditions can cause a lot of stress in the lower part of the woman, so be sure to make a pillow or pillow! Ask if your partner is always comfortable and painless if you have something to say, because you are ashamed, please!

Challenge This is an uncomfortable position (hence the name) and should not be accepted unless you have already tried it in several places. It requires strength and flexibility. Mastery is difficult. safety tipsMake sure the chair is comfortable and balanced. A man should always hug a woman and press hard on her waist so that she stays calm. A waterfall, man, should sit on a stationary chair. A girl can climb with her feet on both sides. He should lean back until his head falls to the floor. In this position, the clitoris is very accessible and therefore suitable for stimulation during sexual intercourse. The vagina has more friction, so it's a better SUV for a climax.safety tipsThis position requires the flexibility of the penis. Otherwise, the man risks pulling the ligaments of the suspension! If you want to know if your penis is flexible enough, press it against a wall. Gradually pull out the penis. If the penis goes straight to the floor without causing pain, it should be fine, but you should always be careful. A woman must remain silent when a man enters her for the first time and inserts his penis into her vagina. Wait until the woman finds the most comfortable position and angle to push without injuring herself. A pillow on the floor should be used to support and re-lax a woman's head during intercourse. Improve sexual conditions· Rotation - in this position, a man kneels, puts his feet on the floor and lies on his back. Then lift your hips so that they rest on your shoulders, head and feet. You can put your hands under them for extra support. The woman stood up, her legs parted from the man's knees, and then she gradually sat down. This acrobat-ic position requires a strong back because it is usually tiring.· Cart: This product gets its name from the feature it creates when couples use it during sex. The man stands, and the woman holds her hands for support. The man lifts her by the ankles and puts his lips to her side. The male is between the female's legs, promoting deep pen-etration and wild, animal sensations. It should be noted that this position requires strength and agility of upper body. There is a variant of this situation called "advanced bull", but in this case the male takes the size of the female and brings her closer to the waist. Thus, a person can control the rhythm of movements, as well as the depth of pressure. · Push is a position in which both partners share and change roles. The girl lies on her back, looks up and rests her legs on a pair of breasts. Walking on the wall feels like getting up. The male in the position of the wall is mainly in front of the female. Women love this pose because it makes them feel relaxed. Men can vary this pose by Kneeling and lifting the woman's thighs off the ground. However, this option is very uncomfortable for women because it is located on the upper back· Luxury Travel: The level begins when both parties are sitting in front of the second rose. The woman sits between the man's legs and raises her legs to rest on the man's shoulders. Both rested their hands on their backs.

After practice, the man pulls his partner to him to find the best angle for insertion. For couples in perfect physical shape, this is a relaxed pose that allows for eye contact. · Grid: Although the grid level seems like a physical achievement. Put the woman in a web view to allow for different types of penetration. There are many ways in which sex can help a man work freely. However, he thinks it is right. The artistic nature of the network helps to create a different sexual situation. However, the system can be expensive or require significant maintenance.· Cancer: As an advanced sexual position, make sure it also requires physical training, especially your arms. A man starts lying when he bends his arms and legs and looks up. A woman sits on it, kneeling and extending her hands for support. If it is high enough, its legs can reach the ground below the person's back. Then lower the penis and lift the pelvis. With teamwork, you have to train really.· Ladder: In this position, the woman hangs from the man standing behind her. The position requires some maneuvering. A man stands behind a woman and extends his hands to her. Then the woman bends slightly over the man's knees and walks easily. They then adapt their bodies to allow the fluid to move. Especially the participating couples at this stage must be firm in their opposition and maintain balance.· Purdy Love: In this pose, the man sits on a flat platform with his legs outstretched in front of him. A woman should crawl to her knees and ride him. By lowering the penis into an upright position, you should sit comfortably and lean back. Take appropriate measures to avoid putting too much pressure on your back. A woman can place her head between her legs and hold her ankles. At this point, the man must lean forward and begin the action.License: As the name suggests, the partner in this article must act as a licensee. The man begins to lie in addition to the woman in a traditional missionary style. After full penetration, the pair begins to rotate like a propeller, and the woman supports and directs it. This position requires perfect limb coordination to avoid head injury or similar events. A woman should raise her legs when she nods. X Shape: This is a position that requires special control and coordination. The man should lie on his back, and the woman should sit in front of him and turn her back. The woman's back should be toward him and lower so that she is lying right on the penis. Her legs should reach the man's shoulders, and her body should relax between her legs. Once the X-shape is finally formed, the girl has to jump up and down and use her legs for more power. The above press is one of the sports that are not considered suitable for the weak. This is a task that starts with lying on your back. As a woman, your arm should support your back and be upright when you lift your legs. A man should kneel and hold his hips, raising his knees over his shoulders. Position allows you to stay still and show the most important part of the moment. By clinging to the hips, you can adjust the speed and position and use them.

Loot: This place offers fast paced challenges, but a smooth and exciting ride. The man sits and stretches his legs in front of him. This position allows the woman to look down at a pair of legs and press her legs against the man's back. Later it lowers to reach the vertical penis. This position is great because it relates to freedom and the ability to engage the arms during the exercise and the biceps extensions.· Fox: Depending on your flexibility, you can go a long way with this position. It offers a deep perspective, so it's worth a try. The man must stand directly in front of the receiver. The woman puts her hands on his neck and covers his waist with her hands. He then helps her put her feet on his arms. During this movement, the man can bend the knee to create a full jaw.· Stairs: The pose gives new meaning to sex and love. A woman kneels on a high ladder-like platform, and a man kneels on small letters. The woman behind him wrapped her arms around the man's waist as they both stared at the stairs. A man penetrates her waist from behind while climbing a staircase or railing.· Deep caressing: In fact, the most favorable form of concentration for men is to deepen as deeply as possible, as this position requires the support of female legs. The female is shown raising her side legs while the male sits and waves to each other. It should bring a man to his knees and reveal the hidden places in him. Check the state of increase: "Not only calmly, but if the mind easily reaches the clitoris of the soul.The long list shows that sexual positions can be diverse and bring new and refreshing results. Trying these methods requires an uncontrollable spirit and an entrepreneurial spirit. However, many tests and methods are the safest way perfection.

Chapter Three

Pregnant sex

Pregnancy The result of multiple sessions of couples in the bedroom. Menstruation can be associated with the need to get pregnant and start a family. Most couples lose interest in sex after conception or when their partner finds out. If you suffer from the same condition, you need to take steps to ensure that you do not lose interest in your private life because it is constantly self-centered. It can be difficult to express your feelings to each other due to pregnancy problems. Sex during pregnancy is safe and good for you and your baby. It should be noted that care should be taken so that no problems arise during the relationship. Therefore, for a safe and intimate meeting during pregnancy, you need to pay attention to the following points. Sexual concepts during pregnancyDiscussion: This is an important aspect of sex during pregnancy because couples need to feel comfortable and relaxed during an intimate session. The discussion should include the issues discussed in the meeting as well as the speed and depth of penetration. To confirm or complete your booking, you will also need the approval of a physician after passing the necessary tests.Limitations: You need to understand the limits of sex during pregnancy. This includes keeping activity to a minimum and keeping the session as close and direct as possible. It is also necessary to observe other restrictions so that it does not affect the pregnancy, especially the fetus. This includes avoiding mixing of anal and vaginal sex, as this can lead to the spread of bacteria.· Recording: When having sex during pregnancy, care should be taken not to cause problems to the woman and the fetus. If your partner has a history of miscarriage, avoid this type of sex.· Prerequisites: If you are pregnant alone, you should visit your partner. That's why you need to make sure that this activity doesn't affect your work hours. You should also check for a history of eruptions that are mostly related to deep penetration and sharp blows. The rupture of the membrane is the result of the outflow of amniotic fluid, which acts as a protection against external factors.· Cervical: You should do a full cervical exam with your partner to make sure it is in the right position that makes it suitable for sex. Ignoring this fact can lead to other serious illnesses that require special attention from medical professionals.Conditions: The presence of a large tumor during pregnancy can facilitate or prevent sexual intercourse. That's why it's worth choosing flexible positions that make your job easier. The black entrance is a great example of an easy and sexually stimulating place. Give the necessary reports: Check with your partner every time you have sex to make sure there are no anomalies or effort. If you experience pain during sex or problems with discharge, visit your doctor. These outflows may contain blood, indicating a serious injury. If you notice any of these problems, you should stop all sexual activity and make sure you take the necessary steps to stop it. Privacy: Regardless of the stage of pregnancy, you should have intimate encounters before, during and after pregnancy. It helps the partner to heal even after childbirth. The inability to maintain intimacy after pregnancy can lead to low self-esteem and, ultimately, loss of interest in sex. That is why desperate actions are needed to restore the mood or completely lose it. Benefits of sex during pregnancyFacilitates childbirth: Frequent intercourse allows women to have more effective childbirth and healing. Contractions that occur during intercourse help strengthen the muscles of the pelvic floor. As a result, the hernia is easily opened and returns to its previous position due to the elasticity of the muscles.· Shorter intervals: contractions cause muscles that help maintain the release of vaginal pregnancy secretions. As a result, a woman may last longer, and therefore she needs less time to visit the toilet.· Prevention: sex during pregnancy is useful because it contains foods from the sperm that improve Health of the fetus and the woman. The protein in sperm provides nutrients that help prevent preeclampsia. Check blood pressure: Sex during pregnancy can control blood pressure. This activity acts as an exercise that improves blood circulation in the body, strengthens the immune system and allows breathing. These are important factors that determine the health of you and your future child.· Humus changes: Humus changes are especially common during pregnancy. It gets worse if your partner doesn't express sex. Because of this, you need to have more sex to concentrate on climax. Sex increases blood circulation in the pelvis, which is important for the health of the uterus and vagina. A mature pelvis is just ready for a safe birth. · Improves self-esteem: Pregnancy affects how you feel about yourself. Biological processes occurring at this time alter the hormonal balance, thus reducing self-confidence. However, sexual stimulation and caresses from your partner will restore your confidence as you will feel appreciated and loved regardless of your status.· Reduces stress: Loneliness associated with pregnancy forces a woman to control herself and take care of the future child. Its most common side effects are depression and anxiety, which can be reduced through friendship and intimacy. By taking care of your pregnant partner and creating better sexual stimulation, you will reduce stress and rejuvenate your mind. Strengthen your relationship: Sex during pregnancy clearly shows that you love your partner unconditionally. They feel talented and appreciated because they know they have a precious gift. Make time to connect with your partner during pregnancy nurture a bond that lasts after conception.evil· Premature birth: there are cases of premature birth in couples who have sex during pregnancy. The number of cases is high, especially if the pregnancy continues in the third trimester. Therefore, you should consult your doctor before having sex during this period. · Genital bleeding: Damage to the pelvic tenderness of the desired state, the tissue in the bed concentrates the male sutures, penetration to or I is difficult. A woman with a low blood cell content may prefer an acute angle of exposure to hepatitis, which is a serious disease during pregnancy. · Infections: Couples should pay attention to their commitment to sex during pregnancy. Some habits can put the mother and fetus at risk of infection. For example, anal intercourse is similar to vaginal intercourse, in which bacteria are transferred to the pelvis and then infect the fetus.Rash on the membranes: Deep penetration and inappropriate sexual positions can cause rupture of the membranes and miscarriage. When paying attention to these options, check for signs of bleeding and pain during intercourse.The best positions for sex during pregnancy· Side-by-side: In this position, the pair lie in a row facing the man behind their heads in the same direction.

This position usually resembles a normal sleeping position, leaving a comfortable and relaxed swelling. Back penetration promotes better vaginal stimulation and the ability to attract women. · Elevated Woman: In this position, the woman has complete control over the depth and speed of penetration. If it is placed on a fake man, the tumor hangs, hugs him and irritates the vulva. · Oral: sexual intercourse during pregnancy is safe because it does not affect the formation of the pelvis. Any penetration is not comfortable for women and can bother them at this time. Anus: does not involve vaginal penetration and always provides sexual stimulation via anal nerve endings. Avoid touching the vaginal opening during anal intercourse to prevent the spread of a bacterial infection. · Even if sex is impossible, there are many things you can do to satisfy your sexuality. A great choice is to use sex toys with you. Your partner may not be able to deal with the pressure of sex, but she is most likely able to deal with clitoral stimulation. Then open the toy box and discover that your favorite mood is the best way to do it. When you stimulate him with a sensory toy, you can stimulate yourself. It is extremely sensual and very easy to Take them to the top.A nother thing you can try is mutual masturbation. Watching you when you are excited is incredibly intimate and emotional. You need to allow them to culminate in a practical way for your pregnant women. It does not press them and they can both have a nice intimacy trying to culminate.Reme mber that when your daughter is pregnant, the hormones in her body increase her emotional level. Therefore, the use of intimate and sensual poses will benefit you. He wants to connect with you on a deeper level, so it's good for them to use places where they can look at each other and have as much physical contact as possible. Another tip for men to meet a pregnant woman, be patient. Now you can change the following as you like. Understanding comes with patience, which is what you need when you have a baby. Sex is not out of the question if he doesn't say it, and he has to manage his own business. Don't worry; Your libido will heal after the baby is born. It just takes time.You may want to keep a few pillows on hand to make you more comfortable, and these pregnancy pillows will come in handy. If necessary, you can use sex toys and grease. Penetration is not always necessary for both parties to obtain maximum satisfaction. While most sexual positions are achievable, some should be completely avoided.· Amount in his mother's background. This is bad because it limits the blood circulation of mother and baby, especially after reaching the 20th week.· Any lying position that requires a woman to lie on her stomach is often uncomfort-able. · And make sure you never, ever breathe on a woman's genitals. This rule should be followed all the time, not just during pregnancy. Sex during pregnancy forces you and your partner to think outside the box to find out what works for both of you. What is convenient and enjoyable in the first and second trimester may not be in the third trimester. You may have a strong sexual desire for most of your pregnancy and then suddenly stop. You never know what you might experience during pregnancy, so make sure you are both on the same page. Suitable poses for tantric sexIntimacy and privacy are all you want in a tantric way. Once you've decided you want to please her in a friendly way, putting her on your knees and sitting down to join her is a great way to start a romance. Your bodies slide together and he can hold you or lie down so you can play with his clit and enter his vagina. Again, slower shaking will help them get excited and learn to resist climax. When you reach the top, stop. Then start again. Tantric sex is about the idea that something is exploding, and the longer one waits for a climax, the higher the climax. Make sure they are both on the same page. You can read the Kamasutra together and try some of the recommended positions for intimacy to make sure this is not central to your entire approach to lovemaking. The goal is to increase the partner's pleasure and prolong that pleasure.Sagittarius: This position is strong and allows full penetration. This allows the man to increase the pressure, while the woman's hands can massage the testicles. Your hips are elevated and you can feel more comfortable if you use a pillow to create the ideal position for entry. Before entering, make sure it is massaged and the oils are easily penetrated. Press your legs against his chest as this will give you more power and control over the process of making love. When you have sex this way, he can massage you, which helps increase the climax.

Making Cross your legs: It may seem like a contradiction, but it got its name because of the area it occupies. The husband puts his wife on the edge of the table. Her legs are raised on her hands, but she crosses her legs before placing them on her hands. You may be wondering why crossed legs are so popular because of the female anatomy. This gives you more control over your hamstrings and allows you to move your body faster, resulting in maximum thrust and maximum friction. It's a great way to make love and something that men and women enjoy. If you introduce tantric sexual practices at will, you will find that you are shy, able to communicate your desires to your partner and willing to listen. He may have a lot of ideas to enliven his love life, but he needs to be sure of his reaction. Talk to him sincerely. Tell him that there are room rules that allow you to freely talk about your sexuality and fulfill your desires. Many women are a little shy when it comes to sex, so they need a relaxed atmosphere to help them be open and honest. This is not dishonesty. The fear of your reaction leads a woman to the bed of the product. Show him that you want him to be happy in bed and listen to him. He may have ideas to fill your mind with love, joy and passion satisfaction.

Chapter Four

Know about Kama Sutra

What is the Kama Sutra?

Many people I heard this word. (This is often called the Karma Sutra with misspellings). However few can define this term in general. They know it relates to sex, but they don't know what the word means.Well, you're right, it's about sex, but that's not the whole story. Kamasutra talks about love and intimacy with your partner outside of sex to make sex more exciting and intense. Although the term is not tied to sexual situations in our time, it revolves around the idea that people are essentially sexual, and insists that sex is dehumanizing and cruel to our detached souls. It takes sexuality out of the bedroom and into the rest of the world in a way that feels underestimated and mischievous.If you're shy and can't do anything in public, don't worry. In most cases, you don't go to the park for a quick dusting. (If that's not your thing, you could have serious problems with the law if you get caught.) Much of your sexuality in your public life is based on body movements and language, subtle, precise, and emotionally stimulating communication. Show that you can prepare your partner for the bedroom, and those around you won't know what you're doing or doing. This is the beautiful thing about the Kamasutra. You can do everything you can imagine and no one will be wiser than your partner.The origin of this wordThis is an ancient Hindu word. It is an interesting fact that many Hindus consider themselves Muslims. Pure and modest men deny their sexual desires. It's the opposite. Indians are very sexual people. They accept human nature, believing that doing otherwise is a crime. If you've ever watched a Bollywood movie, you've seen Hindu women dressed in a very provocative way, which is different than many Judeo-Christian women.See the traditional clothing of Indian women. They often bare their knees and wear sloping skirts to show one leg more than the other. Their upper part, as a rule, is long enough so that the chest is not exposed, leaving room for imagination. Instead of covering their long hair, they wear a veil that accentuates their long hair. They are often decorated with jewelry and other shiny objects. It shows a woman's natural beauty and instead of protecting it, hides it enough to create an atmosphere of mystery and emotion. Talk openly about your sexual nature, but don't get too carried away about night choices. Even representatives of Hindu culture wear provocative clothing. They often wear unbuttoned silk shirts and baggy pants. Their clothes are designed to attract women from their culture. It's all about the beautiful, open and sensual Indian culture. So it makes sense that the word comes from one of the first cultures to use sex. The name comes from the Hindu names Kama and Sutra. A sutra is translated as a line or link that connects things. The range is very deep as it is one of the four purposes of Indian life. This third goal is the goal of sexual desire and pleasure.Outside sexThe original Kamasutra was written in the 2nd century AD. Since then, the book has grown beyond its origins as a quasi-sex manual for those who now want to get out but don't know what it is. faru. However, recent texts do not recognize that this transcends sex. To redo your love life, you will need more than just level hints as you try to complete all the levels and get back to the starting point. It's about finding a balance between your love life and work. Make sure you find balance and not just try new sexual positions. Kamasutra is almost a way of life. Porn is not just another kind of sex .

When you understand that it is not only the body but also the mind, it will be much easier for you to act. You will see that your sex life is not just increasing. Your libido will also increase. You want to go home with your partner and destroy their body, and the emotional relationship you will start to feel will make it even better.Good

! Now you own it. Summary of the Kamasutra. The more you understand it, the easier it will be to master. Advantages of KamasutraEveryone knows that changing sex positions and trying new things is good for your sex life. Yet people somehow choose to continue what they have done. Let's take a look at the benefits of trying something new in bed, including the Kamasutra.Another point of viewIf you change your sexual positions, you will also change your perspective in bed. You can see new parts of your partner's body and experience different types of stimulation. A man's eyes are the second most important part of the penis, so it is one of the most important parts. Women love with their ears, men with their eyes. Men have sex, so they watch more porn. When they see something new, it's exciting and enhances sex.For example, a missionary can only see faces, but if they move like a dog, he gets a full view of them. This is what happens when a woman culminates. They see each other well. Different emotionsIn each of the sexual positions discussed in the last two chapters, the penis touches part of the vagina and penetrates to different depths. It changes the feeling of sex for him and for her. For women, they are all different. Although they are stimulated in the same place, they think about different things. In men, they feel almost the same.· Increasing self-confidenceBelief can be increased by following the Kamasutra. The authoritative book "Kamasutra" offers tips on how to increase self-confidence and gain a magnetic personality.Helping women reach the topThe worst thing for a woman is a climax during sex. Every woman is unique in what she needs to climate, so trying something new in bed can help her get exactly what she wants .Men need to know exactly how their partner's body works in order to know what they need. Cheap. We talk about love, intimacy and practical things like bathing and caring. The Kamasutra is a guide to all aspects of sex and pleasure in daily life.Range often receives less consideration than other aspects of human research. We are commanded to work hard, earn money, find a wife, have children, live honestly and with dignity. But the importance of sex in the human experience is rarely discussed, much less enjoyed. Kamasutra is a bridge across this gap, designed to enhance sexual pleasure and bonding, and encompasses all the other aspects we need to work on with equal respect. Some people wonder if Kamasutra is a truly positive woman, but if you look at it from the then perspective, you will see it as a feminist work of art, not a superficial one.Internally, sexual freedom is openly discussed, which is not always recognized even by our modern social worldview. Try to think about the problem of female masturbation and you will see a sudden clear vision that many people are quick to see. Movies show men quickly sexualized, but female sexuality is often toned or abandoned. This book is unique both historically and in the present because it explores various aspects of female sexuality. Because the Kamasutra says nothing about procreation, it insists that it is a guide to pleasure and nothing more. Talk about overwhelming her with emotions and gifts and giving her complete control over her personal finances.Philosophically, the Kamasutra opens our minds to the needs of men and women and is great for bringing women into discussions, especially at the right time. He has a freer and more liberal approach to women, but at the same time accepts homosexuality and bisexuality.Regardless of a man's sexual preference, it is encouraged and celebrated, and those

who may differ from what is considered norma-
tive do not seem to be judged. The Kamasutra
asks us to question our inner thoughts and beliefs
about sex. Whether we participate in it or not,
it opens our eyes to the many different kinds of
relationships that can exist, both romantic and
sexual, and provides advice on how to succeed
in achieving full satisfaction. This removes the
idea that sex should be repeated and instead emphasizes the pleasure of intercourse. At a deeper
level, this contradicts the fact that physical pleasure must exist in the context of other activities
in the world, and that pleasure is as important to
life as anything else. Life without entertainment
is not livable.What does this teach us? Kamasutra
teaches many things from taking care of yourself
to taking care of your partner. How you prepare
and behave in this world begins with you. It is
a handy guide that combines real advice with

philosophical ideas and concepts. Its purpose is to make us think about what we do and how we can live better. But it all starts with a human be ing.Even if we look only at the sexual side of the Kamasutra, we can certainly see what the author teaches us about physical pleasure. None of us can exist without sex, so why should we minimize their role in our lives? Sensory pleasure is essential for life, so why not experience it and learn to respond freely and ethically to those desires? In addition to the sexual nature of the Kamasutra, it is generally a guide to teach us how to live a good life. It explores topics such as art, music and literature, as well as how to be a good husband or wife. Talk about finances, home problems and choose a partner who will be balanced with you. Describe in detail how to shower and prepare, meet people, enjoy the day and how to please your partner. Philosophically, it teaches us that both men and women should engage in sensual pleasures and that sex is not the only way out for men. Unlike many other historical texts that limit female sexuality, the Kamasutra examines the nature of female sexuality and how it can be satisfied before and after sex. However, this does not mean that the Kamasutra is a very liberal book or that it holds men and women in the same direction. The role of women in marriage was written in the era of caste systems, where the role of women was not equal to that of men. But compared to other forms of literature, it has a more liberal view of sex, regarding women and same-sex relationships, and the idea of sex for fun outside of marriage.How to use Kamasutra? "Kamasutra" can be used both as a practical guide and as a philosophical work. The Kamasutra could be considered as only a guide to sexual situations, which is perfectly acceptable, as much of the text is devoted to this survey. However, in order to take full advantage of the Kamasutra, you must look at it as a whole, consider its historical significance, and consider that it may not be as practical as it first seems.

Many of The sexual acts described in the Kamasutra are beyond the abilities of the average man and require great flexibility. Even the elements in the book are physically impossible if a person does not have a special lingam (penis). Later in this book, we will look at several possible situations and discuss how to create them and incorporate them into your personal life. In many ways, the sexual practices in this book are very similar to the practice of yoga. Spying with your partner, integrating the different levels and feeling everything in harmony, you can experience greater awareness and pleasure. So, even if you can't reach the described areas, train your mind and body instead and try exotic yoga. Since the steps are not always practical, the Kamasutra should be used as a general guide to deepen pleasure. This book takes a lot of important concepts and ideas and breaks them down into practical tips and advice to help you improve your sex life and have a more enjoyable and sensual experience. In addition to the sexual side of things, the Kamasutra should also serve as a guide for dealing with your partner in and out of the room. It helps you to be more romantic and intimate and can teach you how to fully satisfy your partner in a relationship. Kamasutra also analyzes how one can find the right partner based on their personality and attitude based on old concepts and ideas. Although some information may seem absurd in today's world, you shouldn't take everything literally. Instead, you should read the Kamasutra, because in the scene between the lines, even the notes of ancient times are still current today. Sex and moreAs mentioned before, Kamasutra is not just about sex. For example, most of the Kamasutra is dedicated to courtship and love. He says that if a man wants to impress a woman, he should celebrate a holiday and ask guests to sing poems. When reading poetry, people should avoid certain parts. Afterwards, the guests compete in the interpretation of the poem. It also implies that boys and girls should play together, such as swimming. Kamasutra is also dedicated to wedding dates. Finding the right partner is about making sure you have the same qualities you want in a partner. In terms of sex and intimacy, the Kamasutra also includes non-sexual aspects. There are eight kinds of compatibility. The first four are an expression of mutual love, the other four are to increase intimacy and enjoyment of previous games.Palpable hugsThis helps the man and the woman get to know each other and creates mutual excitement, and the man feels the release of emotions, so he starts looking for an excuse to approach her and rub against her. · Obsessive compatibility· Penetrating hugs occur when a man accidentally touches a woman's private parts, such as her breasts, without any intention. By touch, a man feels a strong sexual need to touch his breasts when he is alone in the dark. · Life· AcceptOne of the strong emotional factors can cause friction. This occurs when a person pushes another person against the wall, presses their body hard, pulls them closer and gropes their partner's private parts. Doppelgangers of climbing plantsWhen a female clings to her male, this hug occurs just as a vine wraps around a healthy plant tall and sturdy. Then he pulled at the man's head so that he could kiss him and look into his eyes. Tree climbingThis hug occurs when the woman puts her hand on his shoulder and touches the back of the other shoulder. One of his legs is placed on his hips and the other on his feet as he prepares to climb the tree. Those gestures indicate that he is a kiss from her.· Mix sesame with riceDo you know what a spoon or spoon is for your wife? It's a hug. Whether you are lying on your face or your back, you should both lie next to each other with your legs and arms together. Compatibility of milk and waterSex is inevitable. You will be emotionally attached to your partner. This is an adaptation that occurs during sexual intercourse, when two bodies are maximally pressed against each other, as in a collision. The girl should sit in front of him on her knee so that she feels good and content.In addition to hugging, the Kamasutra also includes kissing. There are 26 kinds of kisses in the Kamasutra, kisses to show love and respect to those used in previous sex and play. Knowing your partner's emotional state when you are not having sex is the best kiss for sexual partners.

Other Intimacy and foreplay include joint massage, rubbing, biting, hand and finger-tipping for mutual stimulation, as well as various types of cunnilingus and flattery.Kamasutra also includes homosexual relationships and sexual "games" such as group sex and BDSM. Love and KamasutraWhen it comes to love, there is a lot to be said for getting it, keeping it and nurturing it. Although sex and love do not always go hand in hand, the Kamasutra emphasizes the importance of love and tries to explain in detail how a person can find love and how he should live after it for the rest of his life. Love begins with itself, only then can it spread to him and to another person. This is why the Kamasutra offers ways to develop our inner passion and desire, but focuses on personal care and personal care. The more you love yourself, the more you can love others, and they can love you more in return. If you suffer from depression, low self-esteem, or just feel bad, you will show it to everyone you come in contact with. You can provide your best version and always remember that there is nothing but hope in life!Love is a very difficult concept, and even if we understand what love is, if you ask 100 people to determine it, you get 100 different answers. Love is defined as a feeling of importance and desire that another person feels, but if he falls in love, he knows that he goes beyond these shallow explanations. Love and lust can often be confused, as they are both trained and played with passion, but the easiest way to separate them is to look at love for a long time, while lust often fades, becomes, or transforms into love. When it comes to love, there are many factors involved in falling in love and falling in love with someone. Love is not easy, it is not without work, and in order to maintain a healthy and loving relationship, you must be willing to sacrifice, sacrifice and work every day. Love is something that grows and deepens over time, like a tree growing from the ground. What begins as a small germ eventually grows into a powerful oak that cannot be damaged by even the most furious storms. But how to grow this tree of love? How to eat without losing weight over time?What the Kamasutra says about loveThe Kamasutra discusses love in depth and focuses primarily on marriage as the best kind of relationship. However, he acknowledges that not all sexuality occurs within the confines of marriage and discusses the different types of relationships that can occur. There is a whole chapter on adultery, although the author does not necessarily approve of such practices. Of course, love can strike anyone at any time, it doesn't always matter whether you are married to that person or not. That is why the Kamasutra ensures that it covers all aspects of love, making it applicable to all situations and all kinds of people. The memorable part of the Kamasutra is that the author believes that love alone is not enough to maintain a relationship or make someone happy. Although love is an integral part of happiness and contentment, it may not be the only thing you rely on for comfort. If you put all your hopes and expectations on one person, you will be disappointed and unhappy because one person cannot satisfy all your needs and desires. Instead, you should see love as an enigma that matches other traits to create a beautiful image. Historically, the concept of monogamy has not been used as often as it is in modern society, instead many prostitutes or adulterers have been used without trial. The Kamasutra contains many references to prostitutes, as their role is crucial for maximum sexual satisfaction, though not related to love. However, because it is not very useful today, these lessons can be adapted as a personal guide on how to behave. The reason that loving women are popular is because they are generous lovers who concentrate on pleasing their partners and have qualities that make them attractive and enjoyable in this regard. While it shouldn't be more than one's pleasure, it certainly doesn't hurt to try to improve and make your personality and traits attractive. We all need to build what we are, trust each other, and feel comfortable revealing our most intimate selves. desires.

Chapter Five

How to Choose Your First Sex Toy

Health is Order is important in our lives. This becomes more important when we are sexually active. Health begins with education. We learn that health comes from parents, books, friends and acquaintances, and physical fitness problems can also arise. But we have more problems with our sexual health. In today's world, the threat of sexually transmitted diseases requires more energy in terms of protection. Whether we play or engage in risky sexual activities, we need to consider our choices and decisions.When we talk about sex and sexual health, let's ignore what we consider fun and distraction. Yes, you did well! Sex toys are also considerable, as this is a health factor.Texts are structures that help reduce the area during sex. There are different types of valuables made from different materials. Marital relationships between them have their advantages and disadvantages. Some of them are considered harmful or dangerous. This is because these things have never been tested as sex toys, so it is not possible to give an accurate comment. There are many sex toys on the market that use different materials and need to be handled differently. Plastic, silicone and latex have sex. Xylin says how are they? There are different types of silicone sex toys in different sizes and shapes, and this is a wide range. They are made of a flexible material that fits very well.Silicone sex in many cases is impossible, so it is very easy to clean. They warm the body and give us a real fight.This is already the sixth plastic surgery. They are usually hard and soft. But it is sexual relations that reach this axis. These types are ideal for creating vibrations and are more intense than jello vibrations in tight places. They can be removed quickly. You can use soap to remove all the blue paint. You can cook them in water or grill them. If you use it alone, without sharing, vaginally or otherwise, you don't need to use products with similar solut ions.They look like unisexual types. But most sex toys are latex because they are cheaper and more flexible than insulation and seats.The best kinds of sex for couplesThere is no better sex toy for couples. Any vibrator, dildo or personal trainer can make love with your partner. Normal vaginal vibrations and vibrations can be exciting, attrac- tive or intimate when used with an alarm. They can be free or maximized in different ways. use your imagination; Explosions are part of the fun. Individual managers must be external, this has happened, and female parts and body parts are not used. These views are suitable for long and luxurious gatherings where you can enjoy every touch and add value to the building. You may discover a part of yourself or a part of yourself that you have previously overlooked.Last but not least, there are different types of vibrators that can be used during sex. One of them is various rings with additional vibration that stimulates the color of women when traveling or rendezvous with another type of exercise. Another has a rotational design that provides IG point and clitoral stimulation and should be used when penetrating with a penis or other type of penis. This guy is stylish. We bluntly, it's not cool if at least three parts are lit (at least you can wipe it as before, but more or less not). If that sounds safe, I think you shouldn't limit yourself, even if you're in a relationship (especially). Discover new things together, discover new joys!At least for beginners with some experience, use plenty of water-based lubricant, and most importantly, don't forget to have fun. In most cases, the integration of the toy is not lost. Leave it and try again later. Most of the previous ones were a bit random, close distances, unprepared cycling, a lot of riding. Most things require some decision. Incorporating sex into an intimate relationship is very different from a free zone. I think life mostly laughs at us as if we are enjoying our successes. Body toningIn Eastern medicine, there is a concept that organs and all body parts are interconnected and that another part can affect any part. Male and female genitals have several typical parts for each major body part. During intercourse and in various sexual situations, these parts are stimulated. This means you can help other parts of the body sex.

The philosophy of the Kama Sutra

As we said, we know a bit about why Vatsyayana wrote the Kamasutra. As for the ancient Hindu texts, we know that four virtues have been widely discussed and written. Many writings have focused on two critical attributes of Dharma (morality) and Athra (prosperity), while a few have deepened the importance of Kama (pleasure).

The four virtues can be seen as the goals that every person strives for to live a full life. There are many references to the other virtues in the

Kamasutra because they are all integrated and must be understood for success. You can't just concentrate on physical pleasures and ignore the need for morality or well-being, so when it comes to sex and honesty, you'll find that they often find a partner who combines sex and well-being. He does that.Understand the philosophy of the Kamasutra. It's important to understand who you want to be. The sexual acts described in the book are a bit more dramatic, with an emphasis on brutal yoga-inspired poses. The lens can hardly be used as a direct textbook, but it can be used to understand society and the individual. Most of this book is devoted to the discussion of the interaction between men and women in society. And in general, and only among them. It can almost be seen as a script that leads us to an ancient love journeyWhat should you do before buying your first sex toy?Want to have more sex, but don't know where to start? This guide explains how to choose your favorite toy for a novice and shows you how to find what you are looking for at home. Whether you want to start right away with a ball vibrator or start with a sex test for beautiful joints, we have the best toys for you with full confidence. Congratulations!Whether you are buying a home for yourself or for someone else, there are a few things you should know before buying a home. When you buy your first sex toy, your budget will be one of the most important factors in choosing the most suitable toy. Starting with less successful sex toys is a great way to expose yourself, but taking advantage of sales without asking yourself if the toy is right for you can be frustrating. Don't forget to visit as many customers as possible.Luxury as a luxury has state-of-the-art batteries. However, it's worth knowing what you want before you throw away the expensive toy that comes with you. We have some tips to help you choose the best sex for your first time!1. Check the detailsWhen you know how big your budget is, check it outVery detailed information on the product page.How to make sure: find its size. More certain than the total length, the inevitable limitation is the circumference (measured along the widest edge of the two). Will it suit you? How it feels to you: The meeting place may seem difficult if the person is friendly enough. Note that the minimum price for most users does not agree with this. This is an additional question. Power and speed: Check exactly what vibrations are generated on the field, what rides you have and how many toys your tool needs.2. Watch the videoWatch the new sequel! Love Honey has videos of their most popular products showing how they work. In addition, it shows how sex works and what it can do for you.

Another good way is to look at a few hands to see what the right starting The size depends on you. You can also get a good idea of what people look like with video. 3. Read reviews However 242,000 people wrote to real people who bought, used and qualified their gender. When we look at a certain scene, we see that there is a certain number of stars in it. This is a trick and a way to see how good the product is and even better stars. If you want to ask me, you can find out more about who I use and howWhat is the best sex toy to start with?One of the first things to consider when shopping for an adult is what gender to start with? Adults come in many forms: vibration, flea rings, sexual accents, male and female pumps, bisexual, walking, and vibrating. If you are looking for the first time to buy a decent sex toy, it is worth trying something modest as a small option. Neither of these two adult toys, such as a silicone ring or silicone rubber, will help make the solution more and more difficult. These cockpits are more flexible than rigid metal rings, creating more restrictions for the user. The size is largeAnother important factor to consider is height. Start with small and powerful forces to gain better combat support while losing more. Mini vibrators reach incredible heights, but are large enough to carry anywhere. If you're not sure you like the Six, you don't want to spend a significant amount of money on your first purchase. Small vibrators start from £ 4, pans cost £ 10 and cola rings from £ 2, so don't spend a fortune.Use sexual lubricantsIf you are new to adult penetration, you can still use sex oil. This hotel is located in a commercial area. In addition, some gels and anal suppressants are specifically designed to affect this type of hallucination and the anal luteal mucosa, so they are difficult to use. Some additional stimuli are suitable for the first time anus player because they are small and intense, but often have a wide range of smooth p atterns.Resources for cleaning sex toysWhen you buy an adult, you should also buy a sex toy cleaner. To buy cheaply, this extra point should be used immediately after applying for adulthood in order for you to be clean. However, an effective antibacterial cleaner with a prey spirit prevents the spread of germs and bacteria and helps keep adults at bay. Why choose glass tiles?The sex toys are some of the best sex toys on the adult market right now. You may think that glasses are essential for adults, but that is not true. This kind of sex object is completely safe because it is usually made of medical grade glass (which is very hard) which is non-toxic and can withstand different temperatures in addition to physical problems. How do sex toys differ from others?These toys differ from other types of toys for adults in that they are affordable and designed to last a long time, while other days may be shorter. Like the different sixes, the sixties can be used in two different addition. Unlike others made of solid glass, it is not used, but with a scream, a knife. Plus vibrations are also waterproof, so it's completely waterproof, this doesn't mean the mind will only soften during the match, but it does allow you to move the planned box of wine once on the screen. Aren't glass sex dolls cheap? To answer this question accurately, it all depends on what you are looking for in an adult. A small vibrator can be a good starting point for beginners because the user cannot see what they are doing wrong. However, smart sex toys are currently limited if the user or users just want to use all sorts of sex toys and continue in the future. For a high quality dildo, start at around £ 30 and can go anywhere up to around £100. But you have to remember that this is not a sexy cup, it provides excellent working brightness, but it is durable and can provide more than one kind of stimulus. They are admired, they feel it, even those with holes and bumps that are often attractive and felt during use. Even the crystals can be washed in the dishwasher!The branch of glass dildos is removedAdult toys often do not open in the usual way. Recently, glass sex toys have appeared, which now have a vibrating shape. Newer adult glasses are available that vibrate when flashed, so there is additional glass to create a subtle vibration. Because this vibrator is almost portable, it can also be used to achieve accuracy during crystallization. There is also no live glass rabbit specifically designed to launch a g probe that has an incredible number of ten different types of extreme bullet vibration. Now you can share!All kinds of sex toysBright sex toysPopular sex toys are "vibrators" designed to stimulate general vibrations. They are usually used to stimulate the colors, but they can be used to stimulate any part of the female body. The simplest are accurate or well-formed (though usually thicker than a pencil). They often have an internal battery (or two) that provides access to a small majority. Sometimes the battery and voltage control are extreme and connected to the vibrator by a cable. This machine is equipped with an unbalanced light load attached to the shaft. As it moves this weight, it pushes the vibration into smaller and smaller circular motions, creating the vibrations you feel. The strength and reason for the vibrational effects drive the search for sex toys.It is better not to be as reliable and fast as possible. The optimal configuration may vary depending on the actual build amount.For best results, buy an uncontrollable vibrator. Different vibrations have different characteristics and depending on your mood you may find more than other and different types. Recently, electronic vibration controllers have been developed that not only provide continuous human / human control, but also allow a large number of frequency pulses. They can be instrumental. There are also types of animated sex, such as butterfly inductors and vibrating blast rings. Other motorized sex toysIn some types of sexual intercourse, different methods of mechanical stimulation are used. This usually depends on the engine, which causes the toy to sexually change shape and move backwards or forwards. The reciprocal movement is sometimes carried out by an air pump. The actions that are created, for example, the dynamics that I like, the vibrations that "turn" the vaginal simulators and the mouth that "works" the man. "Sex machines," which regulate vibration to vibrate and vibrate, are on the rise.A combination of sex toysThat's why we created sexual vibrations, movements and fights. As you may have guessed, they all come in superset combinations.A common combination of many "bunny" style vibes is pure horizontal stimulation In addition. Unlike others made of solid glass, a knife is not used. In addition, the vibrations are also waterproof, so it's completely waterproof, which doesn't mean the mind only softens during the run, but allows the programmed box of wine to move once across the screen. Aren't glass sex dolls cheap? To answer this question accurately, it all depends on what you are looking for in an adult. A small vibration is a good starting point for beginners because the user cannot see what they are doing wrong. However, if the user or users want to use various sex toys, smart sex toys are currently limited and will remain so in the future.

A high quality dildo starts at around £ 30 and goes up to £ 100. But you have to keep in mind that this is not a striking cup that offers excellent lighting, but it is durable and can cause more than one type of irritation. They are admired, they feel it, even those with holes and bumps are often attractive and felt during use. Even the crystals can be washed in the dishwasher! Glass dildos have teeth removed, toys for adults often do not open in the usual way. Recently appeared glass sex dolls that now have a vibrant pattern. New adult glasses are available that vibrate when turned on, so there is extra glass to create subtle vibrations. Because this vibrator is practically portable, it can also be used to achieve accuracy during crystallization. No living glass rabbit is designed to launch an incredible number of G probes with ten different types of intense bullet vibration. Now you can share.Types of sex toys Light sex toys are popular "vibrating" sex toys designed to stimulate general vibrations. They are usually used to stimulate the colors, but they can be used to stimulate any part of the female body. Simple - accurate or well-designed (though usually thicker than pencils). They often have an internal battery (or two) that provides a small majority of access. Sometimes the battery and voltage control are extreme and connected to the vibrator by a cable. The machine is equipped with an unbalanced light load fixed on the shaft. As it moves that weight, it sends the vibration into smaller and smaller circular motions, creating the vibrations you feel. The strength and cause of the vibrating effect encourages the search for sex toys. It is better not to be as reliable and fast as possible. The optimal configuration may vary depending on the actual construction. For best results, buy a vibrator without restrictions. Different vibrations have different characteristics and depending on your mood you may find more than other and different types. Recently, electronic vibration controllers have been developed that not only provide continuous human / human control, but also allow a large number of frequency pulses. They can be instrumental. There are also types of animated sex, such as butterfly inductors and vibrating blast rings. Other motorized sex toys use different methods of mechanical stimulation for certain types of sex. This usually depends on a motor that changes the shape of the toy's gender and moves it backwards or forwards. The reciprocal movement is sometimes carried out by an air pump. For example, the created actions are the dynamics I like, the vibrations that "spin" the vaginal simulators and the mouth that "works" like a man. The number of "sex mashins" increases, which controls fluctuations and vibrations. We created sexual vibrations, movements and struggle, why a combination of sexual toast. As you guess, they all do a great job. The overall combination of many light vibrations is pure horizontal stimulus with vibration and vertical stimulus, sometimes large movements, and Sometimes change is good. Sex can add different textures to your surfing. The vibrator or vibrator may have scratches, loosening or a thin surface. Count on it to get the best toy for you and increase your pleasure and happiness. · Get started easily: When choosing your first sex toy, you should start with the simplest toys available. That way you will be able to work with advanced toys in the future. Start slowly to avoid frustration and intimidation.· Cleanliness: Your body should be clean and hygienic, especially the genitals. Therefore, be sure to choose sex toys that are easy to wash and absorb bacteria during storage.· Preferences: What works for the service provider often doesn't work for you. Therefore, you need to make sure that you buy a sex toy that suits your tastes and preferences.Re search: Products are evaluated and standardized individually. The importance of understanding a sex toy before buying or testing one. · Storage: Special precautions must be taken when storing sex toys. They can react to nearby objects. Often there are silicone or latex dolls with a featured look.· Talk to your partner: For your own good, be honest, sincere, and honest with your partner about your sex toy preferences. Also, let them know your preferences and use their feedback to assess whether they agree.· Keeping in touch: This is an integral part of sex, especially when using sex toys. This way your partner will let you know the zone the toy is stimulating and allow you to explore additional erogenous zones.· Be careful: these toys are best used only for their intended purpose. Be careful when using these toys to have good sex. In particular, problems arise when users do not follow instructions. This tag contains sexually explicit contentAs the demand for adults grows, so does the success of these divisions. People all over the world know the benefits and importance of giving back, but they don't know which toy to buy. This is the main reason why they are always looking for the best types of sex on the market. They don't know there's anything better in the room. Few people have the opportunity to receive a consultation. Others do not.Similarly, a toy that suits one pair may not fit another. Using toys is also an experience. It's a relief, rhyming partners can use toys anywhere. One of the most common myths is that complex sex toys for men are the best products on the Internet because they require a lot of effort. Probably not. Some prefer the common version, while others think alternative text is more appropriate. The results observed using both types are very good.The best factor is always good quality, both offline and online. All adult toys should be used in the exam, and now, according to human calculations, it is useful to use high-strength devices.

Low-quality raw materials made from Эx can be destroyed only by fraction, but in principle, using such devices, they also use their health. Using the best sex strains on the market is easy. No matter how stylish and profitable a toy is, if it's not easy to use, it won't do much to benefit your sex life. Therefore choose a simpler type with a more practical value. If this is the first time a couple has sex in bed, it is more important to stay home as long as possible. That way, those interested do not have to try to understand the functionality of the toy, and they can get maximum satisfaction. *from the product.*

Chapter Six

Sex Toys Health and Safety

The Health benefits of sex toysIf you find them boring, you can find them below. The popularity of these products has increased because they are more likely to be featured on an American television program, as they already have. What is it and what are the advantages of using it?Vibrating benefits depend on whether you are single or not. It's an option where you're in a relationship and he doesn't really need it, but I'll talk about that later. When it comes to the benefits of a group bed, you need personal satisfaction that you can ignore, but you will vibrate more than that. There are many health benefits associated with sex that one can take advantage of. all -However, during climax, endorphins are released in the brain that help reduce stress. Sex has the same effect as a man. Hot heat It is known that good sex takes an incredible amount of breaks, and this is not true while sex does not burn twice as many calories, but it is very painful. It has the same benefits as cardiovascular exercise. Is it more beautiful than a gym?· Improves the health of your heart just as the army is gone and everyone knows how important it is. Do you remember these stress issues? They can help you maintain a good relationship because it can only be good. · That's why sex alone is a great way to maximize and improve your health during this time, but what if you're in a relationship? How can you help?· One of the main advantages of using sex toys as a solution is that it adds another drop to what can be an ordinary toy. Although many of us refuse to accept it, the longer a relationship lasts, the longer it lasts.· Sex toys can help you go further in bed. This spell was not used to induce intercourse, but to prevent them from having intercourse.· They can improve the top. It's hard to understand, but you can find a way to maintain success through a major renovation even if you've reached your fertility limit. Sex releases endorphins that make you happy. Then your partner will associate these people with sex and other brands that you really like and cycling. As you can see, whether you are single or in a relationship, there are no pros or cons to using sex. The biggest reason to use sixes is simply because they are fun, so why not? Why clean it?Some toys contact very sensitive parts of our body. When our fluids come in contact with objects that vibrate or vibrate, the bacteria in these areas stay alive to help our loved ones, but the battery life may not last long.Almost all bacteria multiply rapidly even through them on hard or solid surfaces, and reintroduction of these wastes into the body can cause disruption in their most important places. It is important to check your Sex after each use for the reasons mentioned above. To prevent the spread of harmful bacteria during sessions, do not use them before use (before use in another document) and before use. How to clean your sex toy?You should purchase an antibacterial agent to remove fluids and compounds from the toy. These brighteners are strong enough to kill bacteria, but gentle enough to use after every game.The erotic toy should be placed on the table and carefully washed with a cloth to remove the debris. Then let them air out. The vibration and pain can be cleaned with soap and water (preferred), but be aware of where the toys are used and consider when using soap. Sex toys have a ladder that does not interfere with the child's natural coordination of movements. However, some types of soap do not have this advantage, so they must be thoroughly washed after cleaning. If the solution is alone, read the instructions carefully, some can be placed in boiling water or in the dishwasher for thorough cl eaning.If you work remotely or with electricity, do not immerse it in water, as this can harm you and yours. Wash under running water away from batteries or accessories.If you want to use toys for adults, you can start with a few suggestions:Start small and go slow. Start with a little play and show your loved one that it will bring more joy and excitement to your baby. For example, if you want to try a vibrator, start with something small and dark, like a finger vibra-

tor or a vibrating egg. If you want to test the light early, try a loved one's hidden or concealed hands during the game. When you're ready, work on something bigger and bolder. First, remember that communication is the key to any charity session. If you can't share your feelings or desires, something is wrong. Intimacy and pleasure are the main motivation. It's up to you if you have sexual preferences, but that's okay! Advantages of sex toys· Improves body awareness: Using sex toys helps couples explore and understand their bodies through greater emotional stimulation. Increases sexual pleasure: Combining these toys with sex gives more comfort. Confidence: When you use sex toys, you can be sure that a sexual stimulus guarantees you pleasure. Faster Climax: Reduces blood pressure stimulation of sex toys when a couple needs to climax. Because of this, sexual intercourse begins effortlessly in a timely manner. · Control sexual needs: Anyone can use sex toys for sexual stimulation.· Encourage love: explore your partner's genitals and communication while trying sex toys, remove barriers and connect with each other. · Prevention of sexually transmitted infections: the use of sex toys means that it is not necessary to contact the tool with the penis, thus preventing the spread of sexually transmitted diseases.· Improved performance: The sensitivity associated with sex toys increases the couple's mood, so they act better as a couple. · Prevents unwanted pregnancy: the fact that sex toys do not ejaculate protects a woman from pregnancy.evil· Toxicity: The materials used to make sex toys can be toxic to your body, although there are extreme cases. · Infections: Dirty and dirty equipment can carry bacteria that can infect your body. That's why you need to make sure that your sex toys are safely kept in a clean environment.

The essential guide to health and safety with sex toysOver the last ten years, sex has become routine, and why shouldn't it be? It's a great way to express your sexuality individually or as a couple. Gone are the days when one could not have sex in the unfortunate mortuaries all over the city. Thanks to online games and the increase in volume, everyone can buy and enjoy many erotic games. Despite the growing popularity and storage of sex toys, most users fail to achieve very low induction rates. There are no clear rules, errors or guidelines for a safe program. Many manufacturers voluntarily make beginners and excellent sex toys, and the offer of useful information can be shipped or shipped, and there are many products. This can have health consequences if you do not research. Do you still want to buy sex? tute! Here's a guide on what you need to know to stay safe.

Buy sex Toys only in authorized storesWhile many of the deals on Amazon or eBay are worth checking out, you won't want to think twice before buying. Why is there a false problem in the sixth industry group, especially for well-known and popular brands like Magic Wand? Possible cable faults, underestimating the slaughter and finding a place to contact the manufacturer to determine if they had a major impact. You can never be too careful about things that can take important components and put them into your body. Check your local account or visit one of Bettis Toy Box's authorized online retailers via our app :) Learn more about the toy's features and source here. Determine the most acceptable amount, materials needed and how to obtain materials to which employees can respond.Th ink about thingsYou've probably already fallen in love with this pink dildo, but take a moment to read the product description. Sex toys can be made from a variety of materials, and some are more child-friendly than others, providing solutions for teens. Although cheap products are cheap, this problem is not only very serious. Different products have different levels of ownership. In other words, it is almost impossible to keep many things 100% clean and sober. They are used for all body fluids, lubricants and anything else that is suitable for them, making it a fertile dump. The object hierarchy axis looks like this:Silicone: No interviews and easy selection, these options can be obtained by placing them in boiling water for five minutes (provided the effect is strong). You can spot them with a clean water / aqueous solution (1 part water to ten pieces and soak for 10-15 minutes) or use a special cleaner.Glass, metal and ceramics: These types are very hard, but they are completely impervious and easy to clean. You can wash them in the dishwasher and use white or soapy water.Plastic: In most cases, these are small balls and vibrations. It is best to use a solid, as it is phthalate-free and non-porous. Clean it with warm soapy water and it will restart.TPR / TPE: This is a non-toxic plant-based glue / paste that is extremely versatile. This object is in excellent condition and is certainly more reasonable than repair. Remember to keep it clean because it is a porous material (unless the TPR is installed correctly). Use a fly repellent or antibacterial spray before and after each use. These materials cannot be baked or bleached. Cyberskin, UR3, and other filling materials: Interestingly, only found in Vibes, these materials are soft and brittle, designed to hold real flesh, and have a strong inner core. Because these things are fashionable, it is recommended to share them with the family. They should be explained after each use. The transition between the anus and the genitals is a hug for everyone. To preserve the texture of the bat, place them under the tie and attach firmly to other toys.PVC only: While toys made from this material need to be completely shrunk, the gel material is very porous (especially beautiful) and can be found in beautiful shapes. In most cases, several gels are usually used for their release, which is one of the most important problems of asexual recombination.

Therefore, there is often a keen disappointment, which is the result of the elimination of chemicals in the material. Several countries have found phthalates in containers and bottles due to their potentially harmful effects. PVC is similar to gelatin in that it is soft and flexible, but consists of other potentially dangerous ones. To keep your toy from becoming an easy task, clean it sufficiently after use and store it.

Sex and protected sexYou don't think sex toys are safe to use. Most reputable stores accept that you don't have sex anywhere, and for good reason, you can be sure that's the case. However, silicone, glass, plastic or, in most cases, safes are not covered by insurance. There is no significant evidence of sexually transmitted diseases and the sex you use, although an Indian university study has found that HPV can be detected in many toys after 24 hours of use. Due to the possibility of multiple types of genital tract, HPV, infection, syphilis and other forms, some STDs may be shared. Although most MTS are very short lasting outside the body (parts or minutes), they are still straight. Adding partnerships without a fresh concept is considered a major risk. So if you share, keep them clean and tidy. Make sure the settings are correct.If you've ever looked at a model, you've seen that the installers adapt to some leaks. Real life doesn't work that way unless you're perfect. The vagina is about 3-4 inches long (from the vertical hole to the corner of the plate) and although it's 200% exciting, it has one big problem - the size of your sex toys. Sex toys have a description of width, length and length along with the direction of insertion (how much can be inserted into the body). The penis of the ear averages about 5 inches. If that's your only experience, you may want to think twice before jumping on that 11-inch copy. That's why the very real possibility of shortness of breath, resentment, irritability and burning during sex is more im-portant than you. However, you can adjust the size and make it easier for you to use a lot of oil or a light lubricant that causes irritation. The same goes for anal penetration. Although anal sex can be great, remember that the lining of the anus and vagina is very delicate and full of blood vessels. Fights, insurance, bad behavior and tears happen very quickly, so the best way to get started is to get started. If the analog sphincter muscle is too tight, you can release it, which takes some time, space, and preparation. There are many packages on the market with multiple scoring options, so you can go your own way. Use some of your favorite solutions and offline lubricants. As for women, as a rule, they are not famous for everything. Make sure it conforms to our guidelines. Not all sex toys are reusable. It is important to consider anal sex. Any stimulus is great, but if you're wearing one, make sure it has a flat base or a firm grip. During intercourse, the incredible rectal muscles contract, forcing them all into the rectum. If you use thin and simple to mean full stimulus, that may be the wrong definition. Plugs and anal vibrators are still on the right track. Its elongated base allows them to be removed during muscle contraction. Please, please, never have sex because it enters your vagina. Cover it with a condom for a wider opening, then find a new band for another game. Genital bacteria can leave behind many unpleasant odors. unchangeableIf you've ever watched a parody of Sex and the City, you might think that the biggest danger associated with sex toys is shaking a rabbit. The truth is that some of the yellow options have the ± blade necessary for the necessary and desired AD, which can be called fun - any numbness or pain. Basting vibrators are somewhat bulky and should not be used directly on models for long periods of time.

Another sex toy that is popular but often without warning is a penis ring (penis ring, pair ring, love ring). These are often safety rings that adapt to the rod or veins of the penis and the loom when the seams are not yet completely normal. The idea is to tear the penis's finger to open the mouth of the penis, which leads to a more significant correction. They are excellent when used with care. Although lesions associated with the coccyx ring are rare, they can be severe; This is why it is essential to know how to

use it correctly.

The The main thing is that it is properly installed and slightly increases the control level. It should stay for at least 20-30 minutes. Prolonged use can lead to the formation of blood clots in the veins and irreparable damage. If you are under the

influence of drugs or use drugs at all, it is recom-
mended that you stay away from Coca-Cola. You
can track time and what you do. Finally, don't
stop at the ring.Materials for sex toysIt may come
as a surprise that Title VI is not entirely prescrip-
tive about the type of material used. When you
buy something that spends a lot of time on your
body, it's a long time. This is why I need to explore
what is safe and made with good quality and safe
ingredients. I want to cancel any purchases. How
to do it and what types of lubricant are best for
safety and better shape of toys. I also want you to
have a variety of options and options, so I have
a few options that have bigger holes but are more
complex. If you are picky, product details and
being able to see exactly what you are getting are
key. Now I read most of the time:Silicone: This is
a collection of sex toys. They are temporary and
easy to clean, you can remove them if necessary

and they last. They can be detected using a water / aqueous solution (1 part water to ten parts and lasts 10-15 minutes). You can get anything from a rabbit to a hat nowadays, and I recommend using only silicone, glass, ceramic or metal for the analog dial. Use water-based lubricants for silicone toys, such as water-based lubricants.Lamb, UR3 and other real ingredients: These ingredients, often found in nature, are free and look like real meat with a hard inside. Because these devices are porous, I do not recommend using these toys without using a condom and making sure they are clean after each use. Movement between the anus and the genitals is also a big problem. For a silky texture, serve them with corn flour and keep them separate from the rest. These products require only water-based lubricants. TPR / TPE: This material is high quality, non-toxic and very flexible for radiators / gases. There are many ma-

jor problems associated with this huge amount of money, and it is certainly cheaper than the solution. Don't forget to mention it because it's ubiquitous material (as long as you specify that it's not TPR). Use an antibacterial spray or antibacterial soap and water to clean before and after each use. You may not use or whiten this material. Do not use oil-based lubricants for this type. Apply a mixture of water and silk hybrid lubricant Sliĕuid, such as silicone water, to the base.Lighting and Correction: These toys are certainly strong, but they are easy and simple to use. You can throw them on your plate, take them or use soapy water if you want. Non-porous means the exclusivity of L and COG fat. Suitable for silicone lubricant on this doll, such as Pjur Wome Glide Silicone Lubricant for long lasting play. Jelly and PVC: If you browse our site, you never know what you won't have. There are many reasons for this.

Although the price seems low, the material gel can be relatively pale or Ð bright and s e XTR e m e l ro r® or s, m Á king a BR ee Ding floor f® Rb ac t smiled a. Also many JLL toys are HD. Because of this, many phthalates end up in bottled foods and may be harmful. PVC is similar to gelatin, it is soft and flexible, but hazardous chemicals are used in its production. It is important to wash thoroughly after each use and store to avoid contaminat ion.Use water-based lubricants to control most of these types, but try to create creativity with pointed lightning n and lubricants. Plastic: Often found with colored turrets and vibrato, so it is normal, and because it is normal, it is necessary. Clean it with soap and water and you can repeat. Plastic products can accept any grease type you apply, so don't try excellent quality grease, such as Write Platinum Silicon Premium.

The best types of sex for couples

There is no better sex toy for couples. Any vibrator, dildo or personal manager can make love with your partner. Normal vaginal vibrations and vibrations can be exciting, attractive or intimate when used with an alarm. They can be free or maximized in different ways. use your imagination; Explosions are part of the fun.Personal commanders must be external, and some parts of the body are not female. These toys are perfect for long, luxurious sessions where you can enjoy every touch and add value to the building. You may discover a part of yourself or a role that you didn't think of before. Last but not least, there are some types of vibrators that can be used during sex. One of them is various rings with addition-

al vibration that stimulates the color of women when traveling or rendezvous with another type of exercise. Another has a rotational design that provides I-G point and clitoral stimulation and is used during penetration by a penis or other type of penis. This guy is stylish inspiredIf that sounds safe, I think you shouldn't limit yourself, even if you're in a relationship (especially). Discover new things together, discover new joys!At least for beginners with some experience, use plenty of water-based lubricant, and most importantly, don't forget to have fun. In most cases, this does not affect the integrity of the toy, leave it and try again. Most of the previous ones were a bit random, close distances, cycling unprepared, a lot of riding. Most things require some decision. Incorporating sex into an intimate relationship is very different from a free zone. I think life mostly laughs at us as if we are enjoying our successes.S *afe Anal Toys: For Novelists and ExpertsDonkey flirtsThe flat, sensible size of Little Firt is a sure way to mix (or stand out). Platinum dissolves well in the skin. With an impressive length (3.75 inches) and not-too-disgusting flaws, this plug-in is big enough to rule your world, even if it's small enough for those who don't need to rule it — a perfect obstacle image and potentially a bit noisy. No pureeand useThis plugin is just beauti-ful. It's hard to get there because it's lightweight. Of course, this happens, especially in this style, which is characterized by elegance and elegance. There are not many products that can make this the perfect example for your boat. Because this special rear helmet is available in three different (manageable) sizes, they also took into account the difference in testing and capability. Although this is true, it is still affordable. Aneros Helix SynThe pain and torsion in this beautiful grip has a very seductive romance. Besides, it looks like he came from somewhere. Use it well and send it into orbit. This small mid-level COG challenge is a good choice. You are new or you have known and loved. The silicon in this child is a very pleasant person for me, but the complex core has been passed on to society. hmmmCrystal jelly and anal penetrationIf you want to have a powerful session, Jam (the company that offers the best place for fun) makes excellent anal toys. It has a large 1"diameter and 5"inlet length, a great size to try or impress anyone. You can almost always find jelly on the Internet. In general, bright colors highlight them. Not everyone likes it, but if you want the hardness of steel without the weight (or price) of steel, these are great.*

Fun Amor dildo factory

The Silicone is amazing. it is so. It's good, it's good. This soft toy is a little black dress from the world of the anus: it always has a perfect cut and is suitable for many preferences. It is very versatile, suitable for vaginal or general use. Its delicate curved design allows the vagina to touch the GV or point. in general. If everything in life were planned. Anal bellAnalog accounts can be a great first stop for personal questions. They can be placed on a rope or flexible cable and usually extend to the base. If you're interested in yourself, a slightly broader, fuller, republished commentary that covers a few things is best. Learning to use anal balls is very simple, interesting and understandable. Plus, they're fun. When you start to reach the top, if you slowly delete accounts, it can be incredibly overwhelming. The feeling of openness when the earth falls is enough to ignite your heart.Loss of silicone ringThings are great.

It doesn't matter if you prefer a thesis or several anal accounts can do both. In particular, it has an excellent performance that always catches the eye. They have a slightly narrow shape, which makes them a little slower and harder to climb. The hot topic in toys is real, and these are innocent and uninteresting. Fun curved beadsThese handles have a small gap in the form of handles on solid wire. Being a bit complicated, you can play with those who struggle, but they offer a significant increase in size, which is an advantage of anal balls. Whether you decide to add accessories or more, these anus strips are easy to use and adjust, and are a great way to deal with serious problems.No. Icicles Golden Edition 9If it explodes for everyone, maybe that will be cool in my opinion. Although most metals are significant, these types of solids are more resistant to glass. Are you looking for something with a lot of excitement in a small package? The lighting is perfect. It is very wide and only increases after lubrication. Don't give up, you know when it's full. A large o-ring handle on them will make you useless or favorable to others.VibrationsAll of the above can be enhanced by shaking. Some have multiple speed and speed settings, giving you plenty of room to take risks. Some people like the vibrations, others find them discouraging. They're different, but even if you don't think vibration is your thing, there are great products to try.Double vibration penetration with ball and double vibrationIt could be the Swiss Army Knife of the world. Annual incentive, consultations. Soft silicone balls placed in the mold allow you to achieve uniformity of the filling. Man, I beg, it accompanies brackets and nuts and gives them a chance to overcome a lot. This small celestial instrument has a large grass shaker that slides along the edge. It may not be a fair choice for novices, but for those who know what they like, and for their visitors, it can be a good time. reckless reverenceDon't let your appearance influence you. It sits perfectly on a wide, flat base in which it has an amazing cow pose. First, the tool works, but there will be no answer.

When Curiosity will send you down into the rabbit hole (pun) and you may even flirt with the idea of sex. You've probably tried one or two and are trying to figure out why you've been waiting so long. Important questions for great sex. It's not that important, but there are moments when you're in shape for the next big moment (almost always). That's part of the fun. A journey is a journey. Of course, it should be noted that some unexpected suggestions and opinions will not be missed by those interested. Relax, Dandelion, it's a big world of sex out there!Peridise 2 diable varma Pack. If you think you have everything understood in your relationship, these two will smile at you. Yours and all his companions must be intelligent and honest in their plan. They use their constant, instinctive, natural muscle contractions to create thousands of scars on their buttocks. The result is excessive peak and possibly new pollution. After all, joint projects and hobbies are ideal for a partnership.Friskú annual foxtail tailSometimes you want an animal in your bed. You won't notice the company's signature outlet listed on the price list for the top drive, and the 14-inch range is enough to make fun of and follow through. From an interesting point of view, the code is excellent. Yes, we have proven that the right sex can make you more beautiful and grateful. Combine the two and get credit! Immediately wild moments Punch plugNot every-

one is a queen and that's okay. Among us are, let's say, more capable in love. This is also true. Finding the right items is easy, but thanks to the inflatable game, you can adjust the level of enjoyment on the flight. Using the same type of valve as the Insurance Blues product, it starts well and fits perfectly. By turning the knob, the air is released. Big has never been so affordable .Time to progress!After all, there are many ways to achieve better nutrition. Now is not the time to learn who you are and your role. Take your time and feel free to express all your preferences, and sex shouldn't hurt you. When true, it can be an indifferent observation for us. Therefore, heaven (or your free time) is yours limit!

Chapter Seven

Sex Toys for Female Orgasm

The The best sex toys for female sexualitySome reach the top. Whether on your own or with your provider, the package here at Peretly is fun because everyone should enjoy it every day. With this in mind, we present six (6) categories of interests that will allow you to reach a feminine climax. Really, g-promo or not (we're not human!), These are some of the options that are mostly among us. Maggie's Wand Unplugged wireless massagerThe magic was created. This product was replaced over 30 years ago and was recently designed to make ownership a thing of the past. No, and weld compliance involves variety and intensity of interviews, which is a prime example of a new and better classification. Nothing like that: the cane is a clitoral stimulator with very precise moments, designed not only to carve inscriptions. Jimmyjane Little Chroma permanent waterproof vibratorJimmy Croma, I don't like a set that will last me a lifetime? Soft vibrations are held together, which always allows you to immerse them for some time in hot or cold water. It can be inserted or used externally, and the capital P can be powerful. It doesn't look like Rahalis, so it can be taken anywhere. 4 plus vibrating pairs.Many women struggle to culminate during sex, and until the We-Vibe 4 Plus came along, vibrating rings were a great alternative. Instead of doing it with an antenna or dildo, it's material (can you see the exposure in action?), So she has a constant vagina and a lot of stimulation when she hits big. We-Vibe has exclusive sex with a new level of climax in this incredible position, so it's better than birth. Vibrator Rabbit Habitat DeluxeIn the 1990s, he caused a sensation with his appearance in the television series "Sex and the City". Why are we so focused on what so many women want to have on hand? Rabbit has become a one-stop shop for sex toys for several, and has been a best-seller in recent years.Dan Kush 02 DildoNot everyone likes clitoral vibration or from anyone else, which is why we love the Dantus Kush 02 dildo. They use a better and safer solution, significant anxiety and a little more distance, which gives a sense of reality. The folds are highly textured and the bladder is especially known for elongating the G-scoop. This is a great dildo for those who like to try their luck in the

old fashioned way.Anti-vibration dildo: which one should I buy? Of course, this is a question a first-time sex toy buyer will ask, but I know budget limits and I know your body, so let's see what it can do for you and decide.Clitoral stimulusThis clitoris will help you if a person reaches a climax at this moment - target a painful stimulus from the hand or from its vibration. easier.

There The best sex toys for female sexualitySome reach the top. Whether on your own or with your provider, the package here at Peretly is fun because everyone should enjoy it every day. With this in mind, we present six (6) categories of interests that will allow you to reach a feminine climax. Really, g-promo or not (we're not human!), These are some of the options that are mostly among us. Maggie's Wand Unplugged wireless massagerThe magic was created. This product was replaced over 30 years ago and was recently designed to make ownership a thing of the past. No, and weld compliance involves variety and intensity of interviews, which is a prime example of a new and better classification. Nothing like that: the cane is a clitoral stimulator with very precise moments, designed not only to carve inscriptions. Jimmyjane Little Chroma permanent waterproof vibratorJimmy Croma, I don't like a crowd that will last me a lifetime? Soft vibrations are held together, which always allows you to immerse them for some time in hot or cold water. It can be inserted or used externally, and the capital P can be powerful. It doesn't look like Rahalis, so it can be taken anywhere. 4 plus vibrating pairs.Many women struggle to culminate during sex, and until the We-Vibe 4 Plus came along, vibrating rings were a great alternative. Instead of being made of an antenna or dildo, it's one piece (see the practice hole?), So she has a constant vagina and a lot of stimulation when she hits it big. We-Vibe has exclusive sex with a new level of climax in this incredible position, so it's better than birth. Vibrator Rabbit Habitat DeluxeIn the 1990s, he caused a sensation with his appearance in the television series "Sex and the City". Why are we so focused on what so many women want to have on hand? Rabbit has become a one-stop shop for sex toys for several, and has been a best-seller in recent years.Dan Kush 02 DildoNot everyone likes clitoral vibration or anyone else, which is why we love the Dantus Kush 02 dildo. They use a better and safer solution, significant anxiety and a little more distance, which gives a sense of reality. The folds are highly textured and the bladder is particularly known for elongating the G-sov. This is a great dildo for those who like to try their luck in the old fashioned way.A nti-vibration dildo: which one should I buy? Of course, this is a question a first-time sex toy buyer will ask, but I know budget limits and I know your body, so let's see what it can do for you and decide.Clitoral stimulusThis clitoris will help you if the person is conditioning at this time - target a painful stimulus from the hand or from its vibration. Maybe something very similar to a cock without a 9-inch dildo with a moonhead. Unknown pencil vibratorAnonymous Training Vibrator If you need to turn something on or off, this is the toy for you. I like that it looks like a classic lipstick, and there's nothing about the dazzling passion that makes it look like another "reluctance" on the market. It fits perfectly with everything else in the package and packing in a small battery year in the UN environment. Added bonus: it's waterproof! Let me explain why you keep your taste on the edge of the tank. Vibrator Joben Fantasy Vanity VR12Every woman needs a rabbit in her collection and can be proud of it. He won the 2012 Luxury of previous years and always followed us. Thanks to the excellent excitation-independent motors, the axle and the rotating head rotate harder. It has a subtle curve to reach the G-stop and two test stops to do so. Add to that the soft look and you can take this bunny in the bath and it will quickly become in vincible.Glaciers No.18 Class G-Strode DildoAn 18-degree G-stop on it isn't a drug because before I think I'm fixing the vibration, it's a little fun for you and it's as much fun as it is good. Ice flakes create the most amazing looks with a glitter of all shapes and sizes, and because of their trans-parency, these types last a lifetime. If you want, in the future you can ask for it with hot or cold water. Imagine looking for a mirror on your skin and elsewhere. Add fat and it's magical. When do you do it? The switch is ready! This is my kind of toy. The best sex for women: how to choose the first feelingEveryone wants to know the best type of sex for women and this is a universal choice. But if you've never tried it before and are a little shy, our sex guide is for you. Thinking about building your first vibrator can be both exciting and scary. What if you go to the store, ask again online, return it, and someone finds it? Even if they encounter all these obstacles, how do they know which sex is best for them?These questions. But if you tend to spend time for female masturbation, think again. Each of the six who must overcome these dreams will be better than ever!First, think about how you will get there. Ordering online is usually a delicate process, and it is easy to find out what gender is being sold based on reviews from other users. But if you can't send it home, you can leave it at home from the last place. If you can't order online, it's okay to go to a sex shop. Now that you think about what a toy it is, at least it is. The best sex for women is the one that sets you free. So when you decide which one is right for you, think carefully about how you like sex, and then find the sexual vibration or female masturbation that works for you. If you're not sure enough, consider it. Sexually active women can be conditionally divided into three groups: So, with that in mind, think about what you want to hear when a woman decides she's in the mood to masturbate. However, if you are not particularly successful sexually and do not know what works for you, try not to try all the various combinations, it is difficult. Someone can disagree, even mischievous and scary, and you can start with your favorite toy.

When To make a decision, it's best to start by looking at the best-selling sex. You can do this online, using the books you received, or by contacting the seller. The best choice for women is not necessarily the most effective, and there are many different types of sex toys. Yes, the same price as this is also a new price. As with any major purchase, be sure to research and start with existing toys and less intimate things before choosing a great girl outfit.Regardless of your comfort level, your girls and classmates are just like you and will make sure you love what you have, where you are, what you want, and that you have fun. Sex toys: Use them in these situations for better sexSome points look at the vibration of the company, but it's not necessary. The combination of penis and vibrator can facilitate sex for couples. One study found that users of vibrators experienced higher rates of sexual activity, such as climax, hydration, and desire. Inserting sexual values into sexuality takes activism to a new level. Sexual health means an active and easy sex life, so it's always good to think about how to find a routine. Below are tips for using a vibrator in different sex positions. Of course, groups should be creative and appropriate, but these are great places to start.amount (above)A man can place a vibrator on his partner's flight while waiting. This can be a bit difficult because the big and small vibrators can pick the right way to pick the parts you need.The equipment can solve these problems with a kind of flat vibrator. There are vibrating rings that men can use during sex with their partner, and the ring stimulates the male genitals and pubis. Another option is a narrow room that can easily accommodate both types of couples. preacher (about him)This object makes it easy to use a standard vibrator because the room is more open. He can sit in his free seat and resist the vibrations as much as he can fight and take the vibrations. dog styleIn this case, making clitoral vibrators for women is easy for any couple. It can be pressed, supported by hands or held by elbows. You can also see yourself spreading your legs. The shepherdess is the oppositeUsing a vibrator in this place can be a real pleasure for a man, as the installation of this toy sends vibration to his testicles.free eagleSuch a situation places maximum demands on the female reproductive system. When the male mass begins, the men sit on their feet and bring the girls closer to the woman standing next to them, so she is in a bridge position, only one foot on each side. His pictures are there to get the toy of your choice. a kind of cryYou may have reached a point in your life where you are ready for self-regulation. There are many ways to get a new perspective on life, and you can come up with a new inter-esting idea with unusual toys. Although we may be more advanced in many ways, there are still many self-taught people in the world. The best thing about this new life is that everything is already in you. All you need is yourself, which can be a further incentive.Don't be afraid when I say it! You don't have a ticket yet, but you have an idea to buy. Yes, thousands of doll shops or doll shops remind us of old dark buildings with scary adults. Fortunately, we now have access to many online service requests from the comfort of our homes. A great online sex toy can buy you a new sex toy or love your first sex toy. You can find a huge collection of the hottest and worst sex toys at night to enjoy a lot of things: balls and even men's toys. You have to decide which stone to buy in your world. At first it may seem strange, but you just have to experiment and see what you like. Some small hard plastic vibrators prefer live tricks and try to pin their G-spot with rabbit toys. The options are endless.Now let's talk about different types of vibrations that can be a good choice for women who are trying to get the most out of their vibrations! First, you need to decide whether you want more direct stimulation, G-Stop stimulation or, as the pleasure calls it, double pleasure. From the impressive success of a small group of vibrators to the clitoral orgasm, you will be surprised to find out how powerful and effective they are. Many vibrators are secure and angled, so they reach the inner walls and stimulate the G-spot by directing them directly through the ceiling. Of course, if you don't know what niche is right for you, I can try what I like. Creating duplicates is a really great feeling, and the Sixth Rabbit toy will help you do just that. 'But you remember that you can feel like an eye, not a drain. You may always want to move on to something bigger and better. If it starts with a tiny finger vibration, it's miserable until you think you might have something like a bunny! Take the rabbit for everything!Sex toys can help women to a climaxLet's take a look at the different sex toys and tools that can be used to reach a female climax. Thanks to modern technology, many toys help women easily reach a climax. This section will introduce you to these toys and tell you how they can help you and how to get the most out of them. Even if you don't have problems with air conditioning, using sex toys in the bedroom is a great way to enhance sex. With so many possibilities, the sexual possibilities are endless and exciting. However, the advantage is that if you have top problems, they can help you too!vibratorA vibrator is a versatile toy that can be used for a variety of tasks. There are many different types of vibrators, and let's take a look at some of the types that work best to help a woman to climax. Vibrators have been around for over a thousand years and have undergone many changes since their inception, but the basic use for each has remained the same since then. Doctors initially thought that sexually frustrated women were suffering from this disease, and genital massage was the cure. Although the hands of doctors were the first kind of real vibrator, they were not good enough, and in the end a device was invented that did the work for them. The vibration has changed and formed. It is true that she created a woman for almost two thousand years. There is also a rumor that Cleopatra was the first owner of a vibration, it was a kind of pumpkin that causes vibration: talking about everything that is threatened! You are electric and very safe at the moment. Many of them use batteries and are shareholders. We came a long way from pumpkins full of bees. As we saw earlier in this book, the best way for a woman to reach a climax is to first learn how to culminate. Some women feel completely uncomfortable with masturbation and have never done anything before, and some cannot reach a climax. Some women may be particularly stressed or have difficulty relaxing for long periods of time and have pleasant thoughts. At this time, the hands or fingers can get tired and get tired easily. The vibrator did everything because you could last long after your tired hands and take all the time you needed to rest, let alone enjoy, between her body and climax. Another advantage is that some people cannot move their fingers fast enough to stand up. Others have mobility problems and cannot enjoy themselves without help. This also applies to men who sometimes cannot satisfy a woman without being too tired, or for various reasons cannot have a good relationship with a woman. A vibrator can be considered a tool of housing, thanks to which all women and all couples can reach a climax.

Using a vibrator while masturbating is a great way to explore your body and enjoy yourself. She can adjust the speed of the vibrations according to her needs while adjusting the pressure on the clitoris. Using a solo vibrating session to experiment with different possible speeds, loads, and patterns will allow you to find what you like and what brings you the best climax. Then you can leave the room together and the desired group can play well. Vibrators are used for masturbation without toys, such as exams and solo sessions. Nasr lays him on the bed to rest, arranges him in a comfortable position without distraction, and begins to explore. While your clitoris is vibrating, you can explore other erogenous body parts with your other hand, experimenting with different pressures and speeds. Run your hands over your breasts and massage your nipples to see if that makes you happy. You can move your hand on the stomach, on the neck, behind the ear. You can feel and massage around the clitoris and stimulate the vibrator with the clitoris. Try to take this time for yourself and do it without shame. Masturbation is as good for mental health as it is for sex. Sex is a pleasure because of the release of chemicals, which means you will feel amazing afterwards!The first type of vibrator we will talk about is the clitoral vibrator. They come in different shapes and sizes, and a woman's choice often depends on personal preference. Some are globular, small and cautious. Some are globular, while others are tear-shaped, which can be easily grasped and tapped to access the clitoris. Some are rounded up with a long plastic handle for better grip. They were similar to the first vibrations, had a table at the end and were connected before going wireless. Some of them look like other things you might have around the house, like a tube of lipstick that makes them subtle and unique.All of these vibrators have one thing in common: they are made of soft, slippery materials like silicone, which allows them to slide easily over the clitoris and vulva, and be more sensitive in those places. For ladies. They light up in different directions, but there is usually a button on the side that starts to vibrate. Some have only a on / off switch, while others have buttons to increase or decrease the vibration speed. If you use one of them as a partner during sex, there are a few ways to do it. The easiest way is to keep the vibration on the woman's clitoris while she sits and enjoy it. This can be done in previous games to create mood and calm. It doesn't have to lead to sex, but it often does. You can add it at the end of the session to a climax after penetration or if you are still hot after penetration. Another way to use a vibrator in a couple is to have the woman press the vibrator against her clit during penetrating sex. An example may be the situation of a shepherdess. When a woman rides a man, she can double the pleasure by placing a vibrator on her clit. With enlargement and more stimulation, the man feels this effect on his penis, while his vagina swells even more. This can be done in a bucket position where the male enters the female from behind and the male and female go head to head. A woman can spread her legs, bending one knee, place the vibrator on the clitoris and penetrate it from behind. Another advantage is that even if the clitoris does not experience an orgasm, it will be stimulated by more vibrations, so it will be easier to reach orgasm at this stage when it enters the penis. J. Another way - a male penetrates a woman's clitoris with a vibrator. You can do this like a dog, where you extend down and hold the vibrator near your clitoris with one hand and grab one of your thighs with the other hand by squeezing your penis from behind.Have him on all fours behind you. This position requires a lot of work on the part of men, but can bring a lot of pleasure to women. During sex, you can change the person holding the vibrator depending on the situation in which you are having sex. That way, you can always have the flexibility to go to the right area in any situation and not worry about shaking. If the lady at the buffet puts it in one position and they want another shift, you put her in the next position with your partner and so on. A vibrator is a great addition to a couple's sex life because sometimes tools that help a woman's climax are more effective and pleasurable..

The The next kind of vibrator we're going to talk about is the vibrator. This type is inserted into the female genital organ and vibrates at the G-spot to stimulate her and cause more pleasure. A woman can use it to find her G-spot while masturbating, then she can show her partner how to use the dildo to reach her G-spot, or she can teach your partner what to do with this vibrating dildo. How to create a G-spot by bending the penis. She will better understand how the vagina works and what happens when you use this toy. There is another type of vibrator that can reach the G-spot and the clitoris at the same time. This kind of vibrator is a kind of vibrator and vibrator all in one. One end looks like a dildo and there is

a small section in the middle of the shaft that pro-
trudes from the side. The tip of the vibrator slides
into the woman's vagina, and the protruding part
touches her clit. The vibrator is removed from
the clitoris vibrator and also acts as a handle. A
special model of this type of vibrator is called
a rabbit-ear vibrator. Rabbit ears can be part
of a vibrator that vibrates the clitoris. This type
works because the ears hold the clitoris, which is
stimulated from all sides, not just the forehead.
A woman can use it alone during masturbation
holding the vibrator on the handle to the vagina, moving it in and out, always touching her
G-spot for pleasure. When this happens, part of
the clitoris vibrates against the clitoris. This tool
is also useful for masturbation as it allows you to
examine a woman's genitals and vagina. Maybe
you can't explore the vagina during masturbation
because you have little fingers or your fingers

can't reach the right angle to feel pleasure during penetration. This toy will revolutionize female masturbation and dramatically increase G-spot climax! This toy can be used in pairs. This does not mean that it will change a man's penis, but it can be helpful if the penis is difficult to reach the G-spot and cannot reach the right angle, or if the man has a small penis. It is not a shame to use such a vibrator. If both parties are content, any kind of sex is good for you!Many vibrations are designed to give you more pleasure. Some vibrators have a separate remote control that can be operated by the woman herself or her husband. They are outrageous because a girl can put them in her underwear and take them to dinner or to the movies. This can be a small ball-type vibrator that is placed next to the clitoris, or it can be placed inside the vagina. Then, using a remote control, the woman or her partner can turn on the vibration whenever they want and play with the settings to strengthen or weaken the waves. Some girls really enjoy this because it's just you two in this secret and no one else knows if your partner is secretly in love across the table. Sometimes it is necessary to stimulate a woman who is having a hard time reaching a climax. The problem is that you may need more than vanilla sex, and it could do the trick. Set the vibration to low to give a nice look to your desktop, pay the bill and continue to set the vibration when you go home, turning it off just before it gets too exciting and frustrating. As soon as they walk through the door together, she rips off his pants and begs him to finally have sex with her. This way you will reach a relatively quick climax with a warm, slippery tongue, touching the clitoris as you wish, or moving the penis directly above the G-spot.Another type of vibrating ring that can be used for couples. This guy has a ring that a man wears at the base of his penis and it vibrates. This vibrator can be used not only by women during masturbation, but also by couples for many reasons. First, the vibration of the ring on the man's penis, as well as the ring in the lower part of the body of his penis, hardens and lengthens it, and it is suitable for penetration as the penis. More difficult is a woman's best chance of stimulating her G-spot enough to culminate. Another reason why this toy is suitable for couples is that the vibration of the ring and its position indicates that he may prefer to be sensitive to the woman in the front seat during sex. It's like holding a mental vibrator during sex, but the advantage of this type is that you don't have to hold it, so your hands can do what they want and have a positive effect. Effect of vibration on female genital organs. This causes the woman to culminate in the clitoris and the G-spot at the same time! Ringwave is also great for men, which is an advantage in this situation and improves libido in both men and women. Double regulationDeath is the act in which a woman enters her male partner by tying the anus. This is a common practice among heterosexual couples and results in men opening up additional opportunities for pleasure. However, it is unpleasant for a woman when she is very enthusiastic about the idea of getting this mate. When it comes to the actual physical pleasure of a stimulus, one does not get much. Let's talk about something similar, but it leads to a higher probability of female climax. Stabilization can be done with a double-tip vibrator. Thus, women can also enjoy intense pleasure. It works by inserting one end into a man's anus and the other end into a woman's vagina or anus. If a larger climax is expected, it is better to insert it into the vagina. The woman can control the angle and speed of penetration, allowing the vibrator to hit the G-spot and cause a climax. When your G-point is created, you will definitely connect with your partner interesting experience for him and at home and women, he gives him more opportunities for ejaculation, because you either shake yourself.The best opportunity to study the maximum pleasure that can reach this kind is that a man lies on his stomach on the bed, and a woman slowly and generously puts tremors with fat. Then he is also placed upside down, but his head should be at the opposite end of the bed. Insert the other end of the dildo into the vagina with the legs on either side of the man's body. You can then move your body in and out of the man to insert the dildo in and out of the vagina. You can raise or lower your hands so that the vibrator enters from different angles and eventually touches your G-spot. During this time, the partner's anus moves and stretches, stimulating the prostate and giving more pleasure.Choose a dildoHow do you know which dildo is right for you and your partner? There are different types of bilateral tremor. Vibrations exist in many ways. Some have the shape of an anal bell, while others look like a classic penis. Some people have a system for more pleasure when bumps or protrusions slide in and out or a sensitive area outside the anus. There are many materials to choose from such as glass, silicone or stainless steel. These different materials also determine the flexibility of the dildo. Some are longer than others and you can make them shorter or longer depending on what you like. Some have two similar endings and some have two words with different forms. Some have the same scale, while others have two periods on different scales. Now, before you are overwhelmed with all the possibilities, try to think of this best!

It is a dildo for every couple and every use. In this case, you want to choose the best dildo for the position described above (and others similar), which allows you to insert one end into a man's anus and the other end into a woman's vagina. For this I recommend something with some flexibility, so silicone is best. Glass facilitates cleaning, but does not give flexibility. In shape, a classic penis shape works well for the end that goes into a woman's vagina, and anus balls or something with a classic penis shape at the other end works well.   Lubricant

Less Fat and other tools, a fat lover is about sex. The oil enhances sex in many ways, one of which is that everything feels better and easier. Sex is not fun when there is too much friction, and there could be a number of reasons why your natural vaginal oil is not enough to reduce friction. If a woman has difficulty getting out, it may be difficult for her to wet her vagina enough for stimulation. Also, if a person drinks alcohol, body lubrication is almost non-existent. Female genital warts do not spread as much as alcohol consumption. Because of this, if he drinks too much due to reduced lubrication and increased friction, it becomes more difficult for him to enjoy sex. Maintaining a steady rate of arousal and reaching a climax can be difficult. Drinking alcohol also reduces a man's ability to heal. After all, lubrication is essential for peak consumption. Despite many misconceptions, vaginal lubrication is not always directly related to a woman's level of arousal. There are many other reasons why a woman may experience decreased vaginal lubrication, even if she is very aroused and aroused when it comes to sex. Some of these causes include medications you are taking, such as antihistamines or antidepressants. Other factors include smoking and hormonal changes during menopause. All of these factors cause vaginal dryness regardless of the cornea of the eye in a woman. Lubrication is not just a tool for elderly couples and unmotivated women. Any couple who wants a great climax can obviously use it. In addition to these problems affecting vaginal lubrication, any couple can increase the likelihood of a female orgasm using lubrication. It is proven that exclusive lubrication improves the climax in women and men. For our purposes, we focus on the material peak. Increased lubrication helps establish and maintain rhythm during penetration, making it easier for women to condition in the clitoris and genitals. For a woman to culminate in one of these places, she needs a steady rhythm to stimulate her climax states.

This should happen again and again for the time it takes to climate. Lubrication helps create this regular rhythm, so climax will be easier. Because the oil is slippery and smooth during the sexual activities you engage in, it makes everything look good and provides the mind for movements that are suitable for climbing from one position to an-other. The mind still easily tolerates penetration into all parts of the bed with constant rapidity and without acrobatics. This lube can also be used for male and female one-on-one sessions, even when you are alone, to move your whole mind. No matter what you do, this stimulation of the cli-toris due to the painful rubbing of fingers on dry skin is very pleasant. A little tip for the men who read this book: put some lube in the condom so that you feel comfortable during sex and as if you are not using one. This oil is a versatile addition to any couple's sex life! Next time you have sex, try lubricants to see how they can improve your climax partner.

Chapter Eight

How to magnify your sexual pleasure and much more

While The last thing you want to think about when it comes to sex is exercise, exercise can help improve your sex life. Athletes need to train for sports, and sex is no exception. Doing some of these exercises will help improve your strength and flexibility, which means you and your partner can try more difficult positions than before. The considered exercises are useful for both men and women. Rotating pelvisTo perform this exercise, keep your feet apart and your knees flexible. Keeping your elbows close to your sides, bend your arms and spread them to the sides. Turn the hips to the right and lift the toes of the right foot, the lower part coming out the left side. Then release your right heel, turn your hip to the left and lift your left leg on your toes. With the help of a stick, draw a semicircle behind you and lift the heart. The curve is repeated on all sides. This movement helps to relax your glutes and glutes and tighten your core. It also helps to improve the rhythm if it is done in time with the music. Leave it aloneStart by standing directly on your heels and toes. Put your hands in front of you, palms down. Make sure your hands are on your hips, lift your heels and bend your knees slightly to the side as you begin to bend back. Raise your arms above your head as you move. bending the body, take your legs back and lower your hands to the starting position. It helps open the hips, strengthen the core, hips and thighs, and improve balance. Start in a crouched position with your feet separated by the shoulder width and the toes apart. Raise your arms and then crouch. When pushing, all your weight is on your right leg. The left leg should be rotated at the end of the leg so that the knee is towards the center. To do this, remove your left hand. Return the leg and crouch again. Repeat this movement on the right side. It should be a long and smooth movement. One exercise on each side is valid as one exercise. It helps to relax the hips, strengthen the oblique muscles of the abdomen, stomach and legs along with their rhythm. birdStart in a bent position with your legs, arms and upper chest crossed. Maintaining this position, the left knee of the small turtle can be seen in the hole, the arm on one side and the yellow position of the leg on the left side. ± c step r OC cash ę chest ± open left hands, left hand behind head, right hand in front. Hold the left leg in the starting position, and move both hands forward. Do it to the right and return to the starting position. This is only once. It helps strengthen the upper back, legs, buttocks and hips, and improves flexibility. This is very useful for women as it helps them to be at the top of the page. Great squattingKeep your legs straight and point your toes. Keep your shoulders above your hips. When you crouch, make sure your knees are behind your toes. Click on the heel. This is an exercise. It helps strengthen the thigh and improves flexibility. The last thing you want to think about when it comes to sex is exercise, exercise can help improve your sex life. Athletes need to train for sports, and sex is no exception. Doing some of these exercises will help improve your strength and flexibility, which means you and your partner can try more difficult positions than before. The considered exercises are useful for both men and women. Rotating pelvisTo perform this exercise, keep your feet apart and your knees flexible. Keeping your elbows close to your sides, bend your arms and spread them to the sides. Turn the hips to the right and lift the toes of the right foot, the lower part coming out the left side. Then release your right heel, turn your hip to the left and lift your left leg on your toes. With the help of a stick, draw a semicircle behind you and lift the heart. The curve is repeated on all sides. This movement helps to relax your glutes and glutes and tighten your core. It also helps to improve the rhythm if it is done in time with the music. Leave it aloneStart by standing directly on your heels and toes. Put your hands in front of you, palms down. Make sure your hands are on your hips, lift your heels and bend your knees slightly to the side as you begin to bend back. Raise your arms above your head as you move. bending the body, take your legs back and lower your hands to the starting position. It helps open the hips, strengthen the core, hips and thighs, and improve balance. Start in a crouched position with your feet separated by the shoulder width and the toes apart. Raise your arms and then crouch. When pushing, all your weight is on your right leg. The left leg should be rotated at the end of the leg so that the knee is towards the center. To do this, remove your left hand. Return the leg and crouch again. Repeat this movement on the right side. It should be a long and smooth movement. One exercise on each side is valid as one exercise. It helps to relax the hips, strengthen the oblique muscles of the abdomen, stomach and legs along with their rhythm. birdStart in a bent position with your legs, arms and upper chest crossed. Maintaining this position, the left knee of the small turtle can be seen in the hole, the arm on one side and the yellow position of the leg on the left side. ± c step r OC cash ę chest ± open left hands, left hand behind head, right hand in front. Hold the left leg in the starting position, and move both hands forward. Do it to the right and return to the starting position. This is only once. It helps strengthen the upper back, legs, buttocks and hips, and improves flexibility. This is very useful for women as it helps them to be at the top of the page. Great squattingKeep your legs straight and point your toes. Keep your shoulders above your hips. When you crouch, make sure your knees are behind your toes. Click on the heel. This is an exercise. It helps strengthen the thigh and improves flexibility.

When we Act as an individual and let us express your individual feelings and thoughts. They are detached from what our partner thinks and feels. When we have this, we can stay calm and it allows us to support our partner when they need it emotionally. This will be hard to do if your thoughts and feelings are completely confused. How we respond to the desires, needs and desires of our partner can play a role in maintaining a healthy and active sex life. Once you've been in a relationship for a while, you'll know when you like to have sex, or what your favorite food is. What you will do with this information will be very important.Being open to your partner's sexual pleasure and satisfaction will help increase your desire to be with them. When we choose to have sex, even if we don't realize it, it helps us to have healthy sex. And by satisfying our partner, we will be happy. It helps to feel sexual drive and experience.You will also need a stimulus to react. This should encourage you to focus on improving your relationship. This should prevent your partner from cheating. Sex with them to avoid negative consequences will also not work.Experience and development is what can help improve a couple's sex life. Whether you are looking for a new job or another place, this can help you and your partner. Helps maintain interest. When things are interesting, any couple is less likely to experience sexual dissatisfaction or run away from their lover.When both try to diversify things, it helps to increase the level of mutual interest. It can be a very small or very large change. Whether you're changing the mood by adding candles or trying to flirt more with your partner, you can play an important role in keeping your romance alive. Always encourage yourself and your partner to accept your sexual interests. These interests are compatible with their partners if you have a lasting relationship. By accepting your basic ideas, you can break the routine of your sex life. Of course, this will help you feel motivated and excited every time you enter the room. Another important factor in maintaining the desired level of libido with a partner is to ensure that everything is evenly distributed. When couples are equally involved in their lives, it gives us a sense of balance and helps maintain our sexual relationships. Also, balance in life can be restored in the room because everyone can talk about what they want sexually. When you all make the same effort in your daily life, your partner is more likely to make the same effort. Now that we have analyzed some of the factors that influence sexual drive, let's move on. We give you tips and tricks to brighten up your room. That said, it's perfectly normal for your sexual desire to decrease during your relationship. So if you're taking a sex break, don't worry. There are a few things you can do to rekindle the fire between you and your partner.One of the best ways to keep an attractive sex life is to make it a priority. No matter how long you are with your partner, the room should be warm and spicy. By making it a priority, they show each other how important they think it is. Sure, sometimes life gets in the way, but at the end of the day, we can't let it get in the way of our sexual relationship with our wife.If we don't prioritize sex in a relationship, it can have a very negative impact. Our feelings for our wife may fade, and eventually disappear altogether. It's important to remember that every couple experiences drought when it comes to sex, so overcoming drought and having sex will help them quickly overcome it.

It Act as an individual and express your personal feelings and thoughts. They are separated from what our partner thinks and feels. When we have this, we can relax and it allows us to support our partner in times of emotional need. This can be difficult to do if your thoughts and feelings are completely confused. How we respond to the desires, needs and desires of our partner can play a role in maintaining a healthy and active sex life. When you've been in a relationship for a while, you know when you want to have sex, or what your favorite food is. What you will do with this information will be very important. Being open to your partner's pleasures and sexual pleasure will help increase your desire to be with them. When we choose to have sex, even if we don't realize it, it helps us to have healthy sex. And we will gladly satisfy our partner. It helps to have motivation and sexual experience. You also need a trigger for the reaction. This should encourage you to focus on improving your relationship. This should prevent your husband from cheating. Sex with them to avoid negative consequences does not work either. Experience and improvement can help improve a couple's sex life. Whether you are looking for a new job or a new place, this can help you and your partner. Helps maintain interest. When things are interesting, any couple is less likely to experience sexual dissatisfaction or run away from their lover. When both try to diversify things, it helps to increase the level of mutual interest. It can be a very small or very large change. Whether you're changing your mood by adding candles or trying to flirt more with your partner, you can play an important role in keeping your love alive. Always encourage yourself and your partner to accept your sexual interests. If you have a stable relationship, these interests will match with your partners. By accepting your basic ideas, you can break the routine of your sex life. Of course, this will help you feel motivated and excited every time you enter the room. Another important factor in maintaining optimal libido levels with a partner is to ensure that everything is evenly distributed. When couples are equally involved in their lives, it gives us a sense of balance and helps maintain our sexual relationships. Also, balance in life can be restored in the room because everyone can talk about what they want sexually. If you all make the same effort in your daily lives, your partner is more likely to make the same amount. Now that we've looked at some of the factors that affect libido, let's move on. We give you tips and tricks to brighten up your room. However, a drop in libido during a relationship is completely normal. So if you're taking a break from sex, don't worry.

There are a few things you can do to rekindle the fire between you and your partner. One of the best ways to have an attractive sex life is to make it a priority. No matter how much time you spend with your partner, the room should be warm and spicy. By making it a priority, they show each other how important they think it is. Sure, sometimes life gets in the way, but at the end of the day, we can't let that get in the way of our sex life with our partner. If we don't put sex first, it has a very negative effect. Our feelings for a spouse can fade, and eventually disappear completely. It's important to remember that every couple experiences drought during sex, so fighting drought and sex can help you overcome it quickly. you.

The intercourse initiative plays an important role in your desire and desire to have sex with your partner. If the same person always starts a sexual activity, it becomes a burden. It gives the impression that your partner doesn't love you as much as you do. Thus, the right give and take can help initiate sexual activity, express mutual desire and try to maintain the relationship. When we are young, our hormones get out of control, leading to an overwhelming desire for sexual activity. It's important to understand that as you get older, you may not always have the desire to have sex. This is completely normal and not a problem. Desire is something we need to create for ourselves and our partners. If you have low libido, being sexually active can help strengthen it. By engaging in sexual activity, you increase the duration of your partnership. The only way to restore libido is regular sex with your partner.In general, having hot sex is not difficult. You just have to be careful. Don't be afraid to experiment and try unusual things. Moving from one situation to another can have a positive impact on your sex life. Have an active sex life and open communication with your partner, and you will definitely struggle to survive

Chapter Nine

CONCLUSION

If you are looking for the best options for having sex with your partner, I hope this informative guide will make you a great start. As we strive to improve, your technique is just as important as your choice. For others, it plays an important role in its best appeal (but especially for women), so we guarantee it will. Preferences vary greatly between pairs, so the "best" option for you and your partner depends on your needs, imagination, and preferences. We remind you that you can communicate with your partner before, after and after sex. you like.

Ingram Content Group UK Ltd.
Milton Keynes UK
UKHW020737100723
424852UK00014B/552